Dietetics Practice and Future Trends

SECOND EDITION

ESTHER A. WINTERFELDT, PhD, RD

Professor Emeritus, Department of Nutritional Sciences
College of Human Environmental Sciences
Oklahoma State University, Stillwater, Oklahoma

MARGARET L. BOGLE, PhD, RD, LD

Lower Mississippi Delta Nutrition Intervention Research Initiative
Agriculture Research Service
U.S. Department of Agriculture, Little Rock, Arkansas

LEA L. EBRO, PhD, RD, LD

Professor Emeritus Department of Nutritional Sciences
College of Human Environmental Sciences
Oklahoma State University, Stillwater, Oklahoma

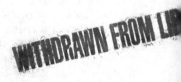

JONES AND BARTLETT PUBLISHERS
Sudbury, Massachusetts
BOSTON   TORONTO   LONDON   SINGAPORE

World Headquarters

Jones and Bartlett Publishers	Jones and Bartlett Publishers	Jones and Bartlett Publishers
40 Tall Pine Drive	Canada	International
Sudbury, MA 01776	2406 Nikanna Road	Barb House, Barb Mews
978-443-5000	Mississauga, ON L5C 2W6	London W6 7PA
info@jbpub.com	CANADA	UK
www.jbpub.com		

Library of Congress Cataloging-in-Publication Data

Dietetics : practice and future trends / [edited by] Esther A. Winterfeldt,
  Margaret L. Bogle, Lea L. Ebro.— 2nd ed.
     p. ; cm.
  Includes bibliographical references and index.
  ISBN 0-7637-3187-0 (pbk. : alk. paper)
  1. Dietetics—Vocational guidance.
  [DNLM: 1. Dietetics—trends. 2. Vocational Guidance. WB 400 D5648 2005]
  I. Winterfeldt, Esther A. II. Bogle, Margaret L. III. Ebro, Lea L.
RM217.D543 2005
613.2'023—dc22   2004018732

Production Credits
Executive Editor: Michael Brown
Production Manager: Amy Rose
Production Editor: Scarlett Stoppa, Susan Schultz
Associate Production Editor: Renée Sekerak
Editorial Assistant: Kylah McNeill
Marketing Manager: Ed McKenna
Manufacturing Buyer: Therese Bräuer
Composition: Publishers' Design and Production Services, Inc.
Cover Design: Kristin E. Ohlin
Printing and Binding: Malloy, Inc.
Cover Printing: Malloy, Inc.

Printed in the United States of America
08 07 06 05 04   10 9 8 7 6 5 4 3 2 1

Contents

Introduction

The purpose of this book about the profession of dietetics is to present an overview of the many career directions and opportunities open to dietitians. This is truly a time when the profession will be what the students of today and tomorrow make it and we hope this book may inspire choices and provide direction for satisfying careers in the profession of dietetics.

The reader will find this is not a "how-to" book; rather it is about dietitians, what they do, where they practice, and what is required to become a dietitian. It is primarily a book for students; those beginning in dietetics and those who are undecided about a career choice and are looking for possibilities. Dietitians or others considering a career change will find information that encourages exploration along new paths of opportunity. Along with careers, we have included information about education and experience requirements as well as credentialing and continued education. The historical development of the profession, the American Dietetic Association as the governing body, and the future outlook have all been updated.

A number of changes have been made in this second edition. The chapters on consultation have been consolidated and others combined. Three chapters have been added that focus on the knowledge and skills that are essential in whatever practice area dietitians are engaged. A chapter on professional development points to those attributes including ethical practice and political awareness that enhance the dietitian's effectiveness and impact and may lead to upward mobility. There is further emphasis on evidence-based practice and outcomes assessment.

Dietitians, through their unique knowledge of both the science and art of nutrition, are the professionals taking the lead in the promotion of nutritional health of the public. Because of this blend of scientific knowledge and social and cultural factors that influence what people eat, dietitians are able to use their skills to help individuals in illness and disease prevention as well as those who are healthy and active. Dietitians also interact with professionals of other disciplines that affect nutrition and are able to blend their assorted expertise for the benefit of clients. Their participation in basic research and in integrating new scientific concepts into practice of both clinical nutrition and public/community nutrition adds an invaluable dimension to the practice of dietetics.

Dietitians are prepared to be versatile through their educational preparation in the biologic and physical sciences including nutrition, foods and food preparation and service, management, and sociology and psychology. This versatility of expertise of dietitians is especially critical as the "global village" emerges, opening many opportunities in international nutrition, management, and food service.

The authors wish to acknowledge the liberal use of material provided by other contributors in the first edition of this book, all of whom are experts in their areas of practice. They are:

Donna Alexander-Israel

Robin B. Fellers

Susan Calvert Finn

Helene M. Kent

Carolyn Moore

Phyllis Nichols

L. Charnette Norton

Sara C. Parks

Carmen Roman-Shriver

Wendy M. Sandoval

M. Rosita Schiller

Kathy Stone

Martin M. Yadrick

We thank each of them for their expertise, their devotion to their profession, their contributions to this book, and their friendship.

We hope that students, teachers, advisors, and counselors will find the book informative, hopefully eye-opening as well, regarding career decisions. The authors believe this profession has much to offer students of the future. We remain excited about and pleased with the fulfilling careers that we have enjoyed. We further hope that many who read this book will be inspired to become the dietitians of the 21st century and help create additional innovative career options.

ESTHER A. WINTERFELDT
MARGARET L. BOGLE
LEA L. EBRO

PART I

The Profession

CHAPTER 1

Introduction to the Profession of Dietetics

"An honorable past lies behind, a developing present is with us, and a promising future lies out before us."[1]

Outline

- Introduction
- The Early Practice of Dietetics
  — Cooking schools
  — Hospital dietetics
  — Clinics
  — The military
- Founding of the American Dietetic Association
- Influential Leaders
- Dietetics as a Profession
- Growth of the Profession and Historical Milestones
  — Membership
  — Registration and licensure
  — The ADA foundation
  — Dietetic technicians and managers
  — Legislative activity
  — Areas of practice
  — Dietetic practice groups
  — Role delineation
  — Long-range planning
  — Working with other professional groups

- Reaching Out to the Public
- Summary

INTRODUCTION

"What is a dietitian?" "What does a dietitian do?"

Recognition of the dietitian as a food and nutrition expert became official in 1917. This, however, was not the actual beginning of the practice of dietetics. The use of diet in the treatment of disease was already an ancient practice even though it was based more on trial and error than on scientific knowledge. Besides physicians, others including home economists, nurses, and cooks were practicing and teaching about good dietary practices, and researchers were uncovering the secrets of nutrients in foods and their health-promoting effects.[2]

Dietetics has been practiced as long as people have been eating. The term itself derives from "dieto," meaning diet or food. According to earliest historical evidence, our ancestors were forced to concentrate on simply finding food with little concern about the variety of composition of that food. Today, however, food is plentiful. At least in the developed countries of the world, being able to choose and eat too much from that abundant food supply has become a major problem, resulting in adverse health for many.

Recommendations about eating and food choices have come from biblical admonitions as well as from early physicians and scientists. Physicians in Europe and China, including Hippocrates, formed theories about the relationship between food and the state of a person's health.[3] Many of the early physicians and scientists emphasized adding or eliminating certain foods from the diet according to disease symptoms although there was no knowledge at that time about nutrients. Until the discovery of the major nutrients in foods during the 19th and 20th centuries, a scientific basis for many of the eating recommendations was tenuous at best.

During the 18th century, research by chemists and physicists began to yield information concerning digestion, respiration, and other metabolic functions. The studies were forerunners of later discoveries that identified the elusive substances in foods that were responsible for many of the effects described much earlier in the etiology of disease. Fats, carbohydrates, and amines were known by the mid-1800s, but vitamins and minerals were discovered only during the early 1900s.[4]

One of the most fascinating accounts of the relationship between specific foods and illness is found in Lind's *Treatise on Scurvy* written in 1753.[5] When it was discovered that lemons and limes or their juice would prevent the dreaded scurvy among sailors at sea for long periods of time, it was a lifesaving piece of knowledge. Vitamin C from citrus fruits was later termed the "antiscorbutic" vitamin. Other breakthroughs came when Vitamin A was found to be a factor in the prevention of skin lesions and blindness in both animals and people, and when niacin, one of the B vitamin group, was found to prevent pellagra in humans and "black tongue" in dogs.[6] There are equally vivid accounts of discoveries of the other nutrients.[7]

THE EARLY PRACTICE OF DIETETICS

Cooking Schools

Early cooking schools in the United States, following their emergence in Europe in the early 1800s, led the way toward good dietary practices.[8] One of the first was the New York Cooking Academy in 1876, soon followed by schools in Boston and Philadelphia.[9] The schools offered not only cooking instructions but conducted laboratories in chemistry and special classes for the sick.[10] The schools trained many of the men and women who were in charge of the food service in hospitals and the Red Cross during World War I.

Hospital Dietetics

Early practitioners in dietetics were engaged in feeding the sick in hospitals. Because little was known about people's nutritional needs in either health or illness, food selection was not a major concern. Menus were monotonous and usually featured only a few foods. One account of menus in the New York Hospital indicated that mush, molasses, and beer were served for breakfast and supper several days a week. Fruits and vegetables did not appear on menus until much later, and then only as a garnish.[11]

Florence Nightingale is credited not only with improving nursing and care of the sick during the Crimean War in the mid-1800s, but also with improving the food supply and sanitary conditions in hospitals.[12]

Clinics

The Frances Stern Clinic in Boston was one of the leading food clinics established in the late 1800s to provide diets for the sick poor. This clinic continues as a leading treatment center and serves as a model for similar clinics throughout the United States.

The Military

Dietitians played important roles during the Civil War and World Wars I and II. During World War I, many served in military hospitals, both overseas and in the

United States.[13] In World War II during the 1940s, hundreds of dietitians volunteered for active service. Dietitians also worked closely with the Office of the Surgeon General and the Red Cross to help train more individuals in nutrition. Dietitians continue to serve in the military services during both war and peace times.

FOUNDING OF THE AMERICAN DIETETIC ASSOCIATION

The history of the profession of dietetics in the United States is also the history of the American Dietetic Association (ADA) because the two grew together in increasingly important ways. The profession flourished because the association took early steps to oversee both the education and practice of its members. In turn, dietitians supported the association and its activities.

Before the founding of the ADA, persons who worked in food and nutrition programs could join the American Home Economics Association and thus were able to associate and communicate with others of like interests. Dietitians were few in number and, although they had somewhat similar backgrounds, there was no way to identify persons who were professionally qualified. In 1917, a group of about 100 dietitians met in Cleveland, Ohio, for the purpose of "providing an opportunity for the dietitians of the country to come together and meet with the scientific research workers and to see that the feeding of as many people as possible be placed in the hands of women trained to feed them in the best manner known."[14] Because this was wartime, the government had extensive food conservation programs and used home economists, dietitians, and volunteers to conduct the programs. At the first meeting of the association, officers were elected and a constitution and bylaws were drawn up overnight. Dues were one dollar a year, and there were 39 charter members. Lulu Grace Graves was the first president, and Lenna Frances Cooper was the first vice president.

World War I was, in great part, the impetus that brought early dietitians together to discuss feeding needs. However, it was also recognized that the services of dietitians in hospitals were rapidly assuming greater importance, both in food service and in treating illness with diet. Researchers were making great strides in nutrition science and, as more became known about nutrients, maintaining good nutrition and treating certain illness with diet became more precise.

Four areas of practice in dietetics were identified: *dieto-therapy, teaching, social welfare,* and *administration.*[15] The vision of the early leaders is evident in that the same four areas of practice exist today although terminology as well as practice in each area has undergone many changes. The first area, *dieto-therapy*, or the treatment of disease by diet, was later termed diet therapy, then clinical dietetics, and now is known as medical nutrition therapy or clinical nutrition. Dietitians in the practice of teaching instructed dietetics students, nurses, physicians, and patients. Later called the education section, this group established education standards and specified the experiences needed in an internship to become professionally competent. The *social welfare* section was later named community nutrition. The *administration* portion of practices became known as institution administration and is now termed food systems management or management in food and nutrition.

The association continued to grow and by 1927 had 1,200 members. The headquarters office was located in Chicago, and the association was legally incorporated in the state of Illinois. The first edition of the *Journal of the American Dietetic Association* was published in 1925 with four issues a year. Early issues of the journal featured subjects similar to those published today. Examples included articles on hospital food service, personnel issues, and special diets, especially the diabetic diet.

INFLUENTIAL LEADERS

Sarah Tyson Rorer was an instructor in one of the early cooking schools and educated both dietitians and physicians in hospital dietetics. She has been credited as the first American dietitian. Ellen H. Richards was the founder and leader of the home economics movement and so is also claimed as one of the early leaders in dietetics. Lulu Graves served as the first president of the ADA and established a training course for hospital dietitians at Cornell University. Lenna Frances Cooper was an early ADA president and director of the School of Home Economics at the Battle Creek Health Care Institution in Michigan. Later, she was appointed to the staff of the U.S. Surgeon General in Washington, D.C. She is remembered through a lecture presented each year at the annual meeting of the ADA by a current leader in the profession.[16]

Ruth Wheeler prepared the first outline of a training course for student dietitians that was the start of education requirements for dietetics practice. Mary E. Barber, 1941 president, was the director of home economics at Battle Creek and was appointed as a food consultant in 1941 to assist with the problems of feeding 1.5 million soldiers in World War II. She also edited the first official history of the ADA. Mary Schwartz Rose was a leader in nutrition research and nutrition education for the public and established the Department of Nutrition at Columbia University. The Mary Schwartz Rose Fellowship for graduate study is awarded yearly in honor of this outstanding scientist and scholar.[17]

Mary P. Huddleston was the editor of the ADA journal from 1927 to 1946. Each year an award is presented in her name to the author of the best article published in the journal. Anna Boller Beach was appointed the first executive secretary of ADA in 1923, served as president, and was the historian of the association for many years. Lydia J. Roberts was a leading nutritionist at the University of Chicago and the University of Puerto Rico. She initiated nutrition education programs to improve the nutritional status of children in Puerto Rico and was recognized widely for this accomplishment. Mary deGarmo Bryan inspected hospital training courses for dietitians in the 1930s and also developed a training course for directors of school lunch programs.

Scores of other influential leaders led the way in dietetics, and additional information can be found in *Carry the Flame: The History of the American Dietetic Association*[18] and in the ADA journal. This brief listing highlights those leaders who played key roles in founding the association and thus were pioneers in the profession of dietetics.

DIETETICS AS A PROFESSION

A *profession* is defined as an area of practice with the following characteristics: specialized knowledge, continuing education, a code of ethics, and a commitment of service to others. Plato first described a profession as "the occupation . . . to which one devotes himself, a calling in which one professes to have acquired some special knowledge used by way of instruction, guidance, or advice to others, or of servicing them in some art."[19] Dietetics, like other professions that fit Plato's description, is organized around these principles in the following ways:

Specialized knowledge. The ADA set standards for education as early as 1919. At least 2 years of college were first recommended, which later became a 4-year requirement or a 2-year course for institutional managers. Courses for the degree were specified and, later, hospital training of 6 months was added to the educational requirement. Subsequent education plans were introduced that continued to specify needed courses. In 1987, "Standards of Education" were established by which dietetics education focused more on the outcomes of the educational process. The ADA took steps over the years to periodically review and update educational requirements as the profession grew and matured. Dietitians and employers alike recognize the specialized knowledge required to practice in dietetics.

Continuing education. When dietetics became an accredited profession through attainment of registration in the 1960s, a formalized requirement of 75 clock hours of continuing education each 5 years was initiated. The ADA recognized a wide number of educational events as meeting this requirement and gave credit accordingly. Continuing professional education is a well-established function of the ADA through the Center for Professional Education, which offers conferences, seminars, annual meeting events, and many other opportunities.

A code of ethics. ADA developed a code of ethics for its members as early as 1924.[20] Updated and expanded over the years since that time, the code is termed "Code of Professional Conduct" and includes guidelines for professional practice (see Appendix A).

Service to others. The seal of the association carries the motto of the association: "Quam Plurimis Prodesse," which translated means "benefit as many as possible." Dietitians recognize a professional commitment to help the public attain optimal health and quality of life through the practice of good nutritional habits. The organization reflects this imperative in all areas of practice.

GROWTH OF THE PROFESSION AND HISTORICAL MILESTONES

Membership

In 1917, the requirements for membership in ADA were lenient in order to bring in as many practitioners as possible. Gradually, however, active membership became based on individuals having attained specified education and practical experience. Several categories of membership have been added over the years, and at present, besides active members, there are honorary, international, retired, and student members.[21]

Membership in ADA has risen steadily over the years. The membership grew by about 1,000 to 1,500 each decade until there was a growth spurt in the late 1960s with the addition of about 15,000 members between 1968 and 1978. This trend continued through the 1990s. In 2004, the membership stands at almost 70,000.[22]

Registration and Licensure

In 1969, the association established the system of national professional recognition by which the dietitian could be designated a "registered dietitian" (RD). The title carried legal status and denoted the professional who met education and experience requirements to practice in addition to participating in continuing professional education, thereby maintaining currency of practice. A national testing program was also developed to establish eligibility. Employers soon became familiar with the RD credential and began specifying it as a condition of employment. Today, 75 percent of all dietitians are registered.

Licensure of dietitians occurs in states in which state governments have passed legislation recognizing the profession and awarding it state legal standing. At present, 33 states have enacted licensure laws for dietitians.

The ADA Foundation

As the arm of the association with tax status identifying it as an educational and scientific nonprofit organization, the foundation solicits and accepts monies donated for scholarships, research, and other designated projects. Several major studies have been funded by the foundation, and programs and lectureships at the annual meeting have been made possible through gifts and donations.

Dietetic Technicians and Managers

The Hospital, Institution and Educational Food Service Society (HEIFSS) was formed in 1960 as an organization for food service supervisors. It was an independent society but closely tied to ADA through membership standards as well as financial support. The name was later changed to the Association for Managers of Food Operations (AMFO), and titles of members became "food manager." Persons completing a voluntary certification program have the title "certified food manager."

Dietetic technician programs require specific education and training, usually 2 years in a community program. As with the RD, the technician member can also become registered through meeting the specified standards and passing an examination, earning the title "registered dietetic technician."

Legislative Activity

Early participation in legislative activity began when dietitians undertook promotion of a bill to grant military rank to dietitians serving during World War I. In the 1950s, legislative activity centered around setting standards for employment in the Veterans Administration, passage of the School Lunch Act, and support of the Maternal and Child Health Bill. Signaling even more extensive efforts, the association changed its tax status in the 1960s to permit active lobbying and made its voice heard by establishing an office in Washington, D.C., and taking positions on national issues. A political action committee was formed in 1980 through which ADA members donate funds and recognize legislators who promote legislation on behalf of food and nutrition issues. Each year, the ADA identifies key legislative issues for particular attention and activity by the Washington office and members.

Areas of Practice

The practice of dietetics was first structured around four areas in which dietitians were employed: *administration, clinical, community,* and *education.* Little was known about the number of dietitians working in each of the areas until periodic membership surveys were begun in the early 1980s. As shown in Table 1–1, clinical dietetics is the area in which the highest number of dietitians work. Although

Table 1–1 Primary Area of Practice by Dietitians (by percent)

Practice Area	1990	1991	1993	1995	2002
Clinical Dietitians	37	42	45	45	54
Food and Nutrition	25	24	20	26	13
Community Nutrition	11	11	14	15	11
Consultation/Business	18	14	13	7	11
Education/Research	9	9	8	7	6
Other					5

Source: Bryk, J.A. and T.H. Kornblum. Report on the 1990 membership database of The American Dietetic Association. *J Am Diet Assoc* 90(1991): 1136–1141.
Bryk, J.A. and T.H. Kornblum. Report on the 1991 membership database of The American Dietetic Association. *J Am Diet Assoc* 93(1993): 211–215.
Bryk, J.A. and T.K. Soto. Report on the 1993 membership database of The American Dietetic Association. *J Am Diet Assoc* 94(1994): 1433–1438.
Bryk, J.A. and T.H. Kornblum. Report on the 1995 membership database of The American Dietetic Association. *J Am Diet Assoc* 97(1997): 197–203.
Rogers, D. Report on the ADA 2002 Dietetics Compensation and Benefits survey. *J Am Diet Assoc* 2003;103(2): 243–255.

this initially meant hospital related, the clinical dietetics category now includes acute inpatient, ambulatory care, and long-term care. The number of dietitians working in food service administration has remained about the same, but more are now practicing in the community and in consultation and private practice.

Dietetic Practice Groups

Dietetic practice groups (DPGs) are formed by members practicing in or having a particular interest in identified areas of practice. DPGs provide a means of networking and visibility among the members of a group. The groups elect officers, collect dues, and publish a newsletter or similar communication for its members. From the original 9 groups in 1978, there are now 29 practice groups.[23] For a listing of these DPGs, see Chapter 2.

Role Delineation

As the profession grew in the 1970s and 1980s, there was a need to determine the actual and appropriate roles and responsibilities of the entry-level dietitian. Accordingly, in 1979, a study of clinical dietetics was conducted, followed by similar studies for dietitians employed in food and nutrition management and in community dietetics. The delineation studies were valuable to the profession because they provided the first comprehensive look at the dietetic practice, and they produced data that was used, with further updates, from there on in the setting of standards for dietetic practice.[24]

Long-Range Planning

Leaders in dietetics have consistently taken steps to position the profession to meet both present and future needs. This has been achieved through planning groups, task forces, committees, and outside consultants. In 1959, a committee suggested that active recruitment, educational opportunities, interaction with other professional groups, and an emphasis on research was needed for continued growth and development of the profession. These goals were expanded in the 1970s with the appointment of a "task force for the seventies" and a study commission on dietetics. The outcome of this study was a report that concerned the roles of dietitians and their educational needs for the future. Titled "The Profession of Dietetics: The Report of the Study Commission on Dietetics,"[25] the report influenced association direction for many years. A second in-depth report in 1984 became a major reference source for long-range planning.

Many activities were initiated in the 1980s, the effects of which moved the profession forward in significant ways. The first of a series of long-range planning conferences convened in 1981 with a second in 1984. Invited leaders discussed goals and needs and made far-reaching recommendations. The future was also explored in a strategic planning conference in 1995.[26] The association moved decisively toward outreach to the public and increased involvement in the policy arena, although the emphasis continued on members and their welfare.

Further landmark studies looked at the education of dietitians, practice in dietetics, registration and licensure, and advanced practice. A "Master Plan for Education and Practice" in the 1970s and a task force on competencies,[27] which occurred at about the same time, outlined major steps toward moving the emphasis in education from content of learning to the outcomes of learning based on the attainment of competencies. A manpower study in the 1970s identified trends affecting the demand for dietitians and estimated numbers that would be needed in the future. Role delineation studies included dietetic technicians and were able to demonstrate what dietitians and technicians did in a variety of settings. These and other studies in the 1990s, including the Task Force on Critical Issues: Registration Eligibility and Licensure,[28] continued to show opportunities that enhanced both education and practice and led to continued advances in the profession.

Working with Other Professional Groups

Since the earliest days, dietitians and the association have worked closely with others in allied professional groups. Mutual interests have thus been advanced and many programs and activities made possible.

Dietitians were initially organized as an interest section in the American Home Economics Association (now the American Association for Families and Consumer Sciences), and joint efforts between these two groups have continued. The close association between the two professions is important in undergraduate education because most dietetics education programs are located in home economics divisions or departments in universities. Many members of each group hold membership in both associations.

Joint projects with the American Public Health Association (APHA) and the American Diabetes Association include the development of the diabetic exchange lists. Grants from the APHA also allowed the ADA to sponsor workshops on programmed learning. The U.S. Public Health Service (USPHS) has established a nutrition section that administers programs critical to health care in the United States.

The American Hospital Association (AHA) is another important allied organization with ADA. The ADA provided a session at the AHA annual meeting for many years and held joint meetings on occasion. Many dietitians have traditionally worked in hospitals, thus providing good reason for promotion of mutual interests and goals. The American Diabetes Association worked with the ADA to develop the diabetes exchange lists as noted earlier. As with the AHA, these groups have many interests in common including the exchange of speakers at conferences and annual meetings of both groups.

The Food and Nutrition Science Alliance (FANSA) was formed with the Institute of Food Technologists, the American Society for Clinical Nutrition, and the American Society for Nutritional Sciences in 1992. This linkage brings together a combined membership of more than 100,000 who have joined forces to speak with one voice on food and nutrition issues and to translate scientific information into practical advice for consumers.

The first International Congress of Dietetics was held in Amsterdam in 1952 with ADA as one of the founding groups. Organized for the purpose of sharing information, the Congress created an international bulletin in 1956 as a means of communication. Congresses are held every 5 years.

The ADA has participated in many programs with governmental agencies including the U.S. Department of Agriculture, the Department of Health and Human Services, the National Institutes of Health, the National Research Council, and the U.S. Congress. Dietitians have served on the Food and Nutrition Board to develop recommended dietary allowances and are presently on the committee to revise the dietary guidelines.[29] The ADA currently maintains liaison with over 140 allied groups and associations.

REACHING OUT TO THE PUBLIC

The ADA has initiated many programs over the years directed to the general public. Foremost among the services offered are the Web site: www.eatright.org and toll-free number (1-800-877-1600) that are available to both members and the public. The Web site is a source of constantly updated information for professionals as well as consumers interested in food and nutrition issues.

In 1957, three states began a "Dietitian's Week" observance with publicity and programs directed to consumers. The effort was so well received that the week became a month in 1978 and is now a significant March event with both local and national emphasis. During the month of observance, media events, promotional material and advertising, and special programs of all kinds are featured.

A "dial-a-dietitian" program, funded by the Nutrition Foundation, was started in Detroit in 1961. Many states now offer similar services designed to provide information in a timely way in response to questions from consumers.

In order to reach the public with food and nutrition information through the use of many types of media, a program was started in 1982 by which selected dietitians were specially trained as spokespersons for the profession. They were immediately effective and soon in demand as food and nutrition experts. More spokespersons, including state media persons, have been added since the initiation of the program. Now called the "spokesperson network," the program continues to be highly successful in reaching the public and has been responsible for generating much interest in current issues with timely and reliable information.

Position papers are another important way the dietetics profession expresses views and presents "state-of-the-art" information in a specific area of dietetics. When a position paper is published, it has been extensively reviewed and approved as an official position of the association. Position papers are widely used and often quoted by the media and are used in legislative activities. Each paper is reviewed on a regular basis for currency of information to reflect the most scientifically accurate views.

Participation in national projects and campaigns is another way the association impacts the public. Over the years, campaigns for women's health, child nutrition, osteoporosis, high blood pressure, and others have been the focus of several medical and health-related groups including the ADA. The national effort to improve the health of the nation is centered in the "Healthy People 2010" campaign currently underway by the National Institutes of Health.[30] The goals are updated every 10 years and list a broad range of health-related conditions and practices in the United States that require attention and improvement. In part because of the participation of professional groups and governmental agencies, this is a program with far-reaching impact for the public.

SUMMARY

The past history of the dietetics profession is a rich account of consistent growth, forward-thinking leaders, and the recognition of dietitians as leaders among those concerned with the health and well-being of all citizens. As a profession, dietetics has established standards for education of practitioners, a code of ethics, registration and licensure, and a tradition of joining forces with others in allied areas of professional practice to extend outreach and service. The ADA stands for and supports its members as they practice in a wide variety of careers and also reaches out to the public with timely and reliable information about food and nutrition issues.

DEFINITIONS

The American Dietetic Association (ADA). The professional organization for dietitians.

The American Dietetic Association Foundation (ADAF). The arm of the association with a tax status enabling acceptance of funds for designated purposes of benefit to the association and the public.

Dietetic Practice Group (DPG). Organized group of dietitians with similar interests in an area of practice or a particular subject area.

Dietetic Technician. Graduate of an approved dietetic technician program.

Dietitian. A professional who translates the science of food and nutrition to enhance the health and well-being of individuals and groups.

Licensed Dietitian (LD). A dietitian meeting the credentialing requirements of a state to engage in the practice of dietetics.

Nutritionist. A professional with academic credentials in nutrition; may also be an RD.

Professional. A person who has attained specialized knowledge and high standards of commitment in an area of practice.

Quality Assurance. Certification of the continuous, optimal, effective, and efficient outcomes of a service or program.

Registered Dietitian (RD). A dietitian meeting the eligibility requirements of the Commission on Dietetic Registration.

Role Delineation. A study of the levels of involvement in activities and roles of practitioners.

Standards of Practice. Statements of the practitioner's responsibility for providing quality nutrition care or other designated responsibilities according to the area of practice.

REFERENCES

1. Barber, M.I. *History of the American Dietetic Association (1917–1959)*. Philadelphia: JB Lippincott Co., 1959.
2. Corbett, F.R. "The Training of Dietitians for Hospitals." *J Home Ec* 1(1909): 62.

3. ADA. *A New Look at the Profession of Dietetics. Report of the 1984 Study Commission on Dietetics.* Chicago: The American Dietetic Association, 1985.

4. Todhunter, E.N. "Development of Knowledge in Nutrition. I. Animal experiments." *J Am Diet Assoc* 41(1962): 328–334.

5. Beeuwkes, A.M. "The Prevalence of Scurvy among Voyageurs to America 1493–1600." *J Am Diet Assoc* 24(1948): 300–303.

6. Goldberger, J. "Pellagra." *J Am Diet Assoc* 4(1929): 221–227.

7. McCoy, C.M. "Seven Centuries of Scientific Nutrition." *J Am Diet Assoc* 15(1939): 648–658.

8. Shircliffe, A. "American Schools of Cookery." *J Am Diet Assoc* 23(1947): 776–777.

9. See Note 3.

10. Rorer, S.T. "Early Dietetics." *J Am Diet Assoc* 10(1934): 289–295.

11. Cassell, J. *Carry the Flame: The History of the American Dietetic Association.* Chicago: The American Dietetic Association, 1990.

12. Cooper, L.F. "Florence Nightingale's Contribution to Dietetics." *J Am Diet Assoc* 30(1954): 121–127.

13. See Note 10.

14. See Note 11.

15. See Note 3.

16. See Note 11.

17. Ibid.

18. Ibid.

19. See Note 5.

20. See Note 11.

21. Bylaws of the American Dietetic Association. Chicago. Revised March 2003.

22. Personal Communication. Karen Lechowich, American Dietetic Association, Chicago, 2004.

23. The American Dietetic Association. "2003–2004 Dietetic Practice Groups." www.eatright.org (accessed March 1, 2004).

24. Kane, M.T., C.A. Estes, D.A. Colton, and C.S. Eltoft. "Role Delineation for Dietetic Practitioners: Empirical Results." *J Am Diet Assoc* 90(1990): 1124–1133.

25. ADA. *The Profession of Dietetics: The Report of the Study Commission on Dietetics.* Chicago: The American Dietetic Association, 1972.

26. ADA. *ADA Annual Report, 1994–1995.* Chicago: The American Dietetic Association; 1995.

27. Council on Educational Preparation. "Report of the Task Force on Competencies." *J Am Diet Assoc* 73(1978): 281.

28. ADA. *Report of the Critical Issues: Registration Eligibility and Licensure Task Force.* Chicago: The American Dietetic Association; 1992.

29. The American Dietetic Association. "Five Members on New Dietary Guidelines and Food Guide Pyramid Advisory Committee." *ADA Times* 1, no. 2(November–December 2002): 2.

30. *Healthy People 2010. Understanding and Improving Health.* National Institutes of Health, 2000.

CHAPTER 2

The American Dietetic Association

"In the history of the dietetics profession, there have never been more diverse or more interesting opportunities for dietitians and dietetic technicians. New levels of competence will continue to open doors in food and nutrition areas."[1]

Outline

- Introduction
- The Strategic Plan
- Membership Categories
- Benefits of Membership
- Governance of the Association
  - Board of directors (BOD)
  - House of delegates (HOD)
  - Commission on accreditation for dietetics education (CADE)
  - Commission on dietetic registration (CDR)
  - Dietetic practice groups (DPGs)
  - Standards of professional practice
  - Position papers
  - Professional code of ethics
  - Salaries
- Affiliated Units of the American Dietetic Association
  - State and district associations
  - American dietetic association foundation
  - Washington office
- Summary

INTRODUCTION

The American Dietetic Association (ADA), formed by a small group of dietitians in 1917, stands as the professional organization of nearly 70,000 food and nutrition experts. In the 80-plus years since its founding, the association has been the major forum for the networking of dietitians, presentation of research related to food and nutrition, and the political activities necessary to govern this large organization.

Although the original constitution and bylaws of the association have been amended frequently, the focus of the association has remained constant from the beginning: maintaining a concern for the continuing interest of dietitians and dietetic professionals in their education, practice opportunities, and research for the future. The ADA and the profession of dietetics have become almost synonymous. This clearly shows the long-standing concerns of the two groups as similar protection of the public in areas of nutritional health and disease prevention and the welfare of the practitioner (or individual member). The organization of the association and the leadership of elected members have worked through the years to keep these concerns in focus.

Part of the mission statement of ADA says: "leading the future of dietetics." This mission statement sets the agenda of the association and its programs. The vision of the association declares that "American Dietetic Association members are the most valued source of food and nutrition services." This vision delineates the responsibility of each member to the highest professional standards of practice and sets the stage for the agreed-on values: *customer focus, integrity, innovation, life-long learning, collaboration, inclusivity, and social responsibility*. These values are defined here[2]:

Customer focus—operates with consideration for the needs and expectations of internal and external customers.

Integrity—acts ethically, with accountability and attention to excellence.

Innovation—fosters an environment of positive change through creative and continuous improvement.

Life-long learning—takes personal accountability for own competence, seeks opportunities for continued learning.

Collaboration—promotes open dialogue, cooperation, and the sharing of knowledge.

Inclusivity—demonstrates respect and sensitivity toward and appreciation of the backgrounds, differences, and points of view of others.

Social responsibility—guides decisions and actions by considering economic, environmental, and social implications.

THE STRATEGIC PLAN

Through activation of the mission and vision statements along with the goals for action, a strategic plan for the association and its members is in effect. Six major goals are identified in the strategic plan (see Figure 2–1)[3]:

1. *To increase demand and utilization of services provided by members.*
2. *Empower members to compete successfully in a rapidly changing environment.*
3. *Proactively focus on emerging areas of food and nutrition.*
4. *Build an aligned, engaged, and diverse membership.*
5. *Influence key food, nutrition, and health initiatives.*
6. *Impact the research agenda and facilitate research supporting the dietetics profession.*

MEMBERSHIP CATEGORIES

Membership in the ADA is available in the categories of active, honorary, retired, and student (see Appendix B). The largest category is *active,* which, in general, includes those who hold a baccalaureate degree and have met academic requirements specified by the ADA; an individual with an advanced degree and an emphasis in a closely allied area with dietetics; or a registered dietetic technician (DTR). In addition, any person who has completed a term as president of the association or one who has previously paid dues to obtain "life membership" may also be considered as active members.

The *retired* member category is an option for any member who is at least 62 years of age, either actively employed or no longer employed. *Student* members are those enrolled in an accredited program, a student in a college degree program intending to enter an accredited program, or active members returning to school for a degree in a dietetic-related course of study. *Honorary* membership is awarded to individuals who have made contributions to the field of nutrition or dietetics and are deemed eligible by the board of directors. *International* members are those persons who have completed formal training outside the United States and U.S. territories and have been verified by a country's professional dietetics association or regulatory body.

The rights and privileges of each of the membership categories appear in the bylaws of ADA (see www.eatright.org). The dues may change from year to year by action of the house of delegates. Those interested should review the current bylaws of the association for additional details. Dues are different for each category, with a portion of the national dues offsetting the cost of the *Journal of the American Dietetic Association* and a rebate returned to the state affiliate association for each

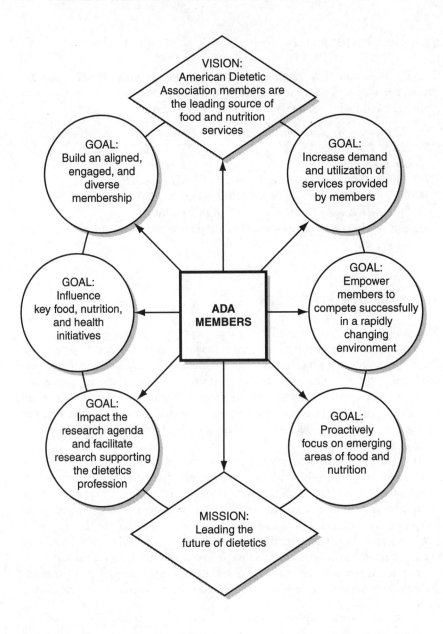

Figure 2–1   Strategic Planning Task Force Recommendations. *Source:* ADA. "Strategic Plan 2003." www.eatright.org/member/governance (accessed February 28, 2004).

member from that state. In addition, the national dietetic practice groups (DPGs) charge for membership in their groups and provide newsletters and other educational materials for members in the specific practice areas.

BENEFITS OF MEMBERSHIP

Membership in the association benefits the individual and collective members in many ways. For example:

- quality standards for entry-level education
- 29 practice groups for networking in specific areas of practice
- positions on food and nutrition issues
- an annual meeting and exhibition showcasing the latest in technology and products
- credentialing programs for various levels of practice
- a peer-reviewed respected journal; the *Journal of the American Dietetic Association*
- educational materials for use in the practice of dietetics
- access to professional education opportunities
- collaboration with international groups promoting global nutrition activities
- scholarships and research funding through the ADA Foundation

GOVERNANCE OF THE ASSOCIATION

The organizational structure of the association has changed over time; however, in general, the governance has been through volunteers who are elected from the membership-at-large to serve on the board of directors (BOD). A chief executive officer (CEO) is employed by the board to oversee and manage a paid staff at the headquarters office in Chicago. Under the leadership of the chief operating officer, the paid staff form partnerships with the various volunteer groups, forming teams to accomplish the variety of tasks necessary to keep the organization functional and to implement the strategic plan. The BOD governs the organization through the elected officers of the association, and the house of delegates (HOD) governs the profession, functioning as a voice for members.

Board of Directors (BOD)

The BOD is composed of 18 members: president, president-elect, past president, treasurer, treasurer-elect, three directors at large, six HOD directors, two public members, the ADA Foundation chair, and the CEO of ADA who is ex-officio. The BOD governs the organization through the following activities:

- sets and monitors strategic direction
- oversees fiscal planning
- provides leadership for professional initiatives
- selects, supports, and assesses the CEO and conducts an annual performance appraisal
- appoints persons to represent the association
- establishes guidelines and policies for appeals, publications, awards, and honors
- administers and enforces the professional code of ethics
- exercises powers and performs lawful acts under the Illinois Not-for-Profit Corporation Act

House of Delegates (HOD)

The HOD is composed of 110 affiliate delegates representing the 53 affiliate dietetic associations and elected by the affiliate members. In addition, there are 18 "professional issues" delegates representing the DPGs who are elected by the general ADA membership. Ten at-large delegates are also in the house, representing groups as follows: one from the Commission on Accreditation for Dietetics Education (CADE), one delegate representing the Commission on Dietetic Registration, two delegates from the DTR, one representing student members, one representing retired members, one representing members under 30 years of age, three delegates from the broad membership, and finally, six HOD directors who comprise the house leadership team and who are elected by the BOD.

The HOD has the following responsibilities toward governing the profession:

- adopts and revises with the Commission on Dietetic Registration (CDR) a code of ethics for dietetic practitioners, disciplinary procedures for unethical conduct, and reinstatement conditions
- makes recommendations on standards, qualifications, and other issues related to credentialing to the CDR
- makes recommendations on accreditation and related issues to the CADE
- provides direction for quality management in dietetic practice
- identifies and develops position statements
- provides oversight to ADA and affiliate bylaws
- assists with recruitment and retention efforts related to leadership development

Both the BOD and the HOD represent ADA members and govern the profession. As a comparison, the BOD is likened to the executive branch and the HOD the legislative branch. Both groups work closely to promote the interest of the members and further the profession.

Commission on Accreditation for Dietetics Education (CADE)

The CADE establishes and enforces standards for the educational preparation of dietetics professionals and recognized dietetics education programs that meet the standards. The CADE administers and has authority for all actions that apply to accreditation of entry-level education programs that include standard setting, fees, finances, and administration. There are 12 members on the commission. At least half the members represent each program type (dietetic technician, didactic, coordinated, and dietetic internship). The commission includes one representative of other constituents, a dietetic student, and two representatives of the public.

Commission on Dietetic Registration (CDR)

The CDR sets the standards for certification and recertification and enforces the code of ethics of the association. The commission issues credentials to those individuals who meet the standards. Dietitians thus attain the Registered Dietitian designation and the DTR. Specialists receive the certified specialist title (see Chapter 4).

Dietetic Practice Groups (DPGs)

The practice groups are professional interest groups within the ADA framework. There are 29 active groups and they show the diversity of the practice areas in which dietitians work (Table 2–1). Each of the groups networks to serve its members, charges fees to support its activities, and publishes periodic newsletters. The groups also sponsor educational sessions at the annual meeting of ADA. The only requirement to join a DPG is ADA membership or registration status and the payment of dues.

Formation of new DPGs occurs after interest groups become large enough to seek official status. A petition is submitted with no less than 500 signatures indicating interest and individuals willing to serve as officers, plus a budget. Aside from maintaining a minimum (300) of members, other uniform requirements include publication of a newsletter at least quarterly for its members, maintaining governing documents, conducting an annual meeting of its members, and maintaining a

Table 2–1   Dietetic Practice Groups 2003–2004

Dietetic Practice Group	Description
Clinical Nutrition Management DPG	Managers who direct clinical nutrition programs across the continuum of care.
Consultant Dietitians in Health Care Facilities	Practitioners typically employed under contract who provide nutrition consultation to acute and long-term-care facilities, home care companies, health care agencies, and the food service industry.
Diabetes Care and Education (DCE) DPG	Members involved in patient education, professional education, and research for the management of diabetes mellitus.
Dietetic Educators of Practitioners (DEP) DPG	Educators of dietetics practitioners for entry and advanced levels of dietetics practice.
Dietetic Technicians in Practice DPG	Dietetic technicians, dietetic technician educators, and dietetic technician employers who focus on the competencies, skills, and needs of dietetic technicians.
Dietetics in Developmental and Psychiatric Disorders DPG	Nutrition professionals whose work involves clients with physical and mental disabilities, developmental disorders, psychiatric illnesses, substance abuse problems, and eating disorders.
Dietetics in Physical Medicine and Rehabilitation DPG	Practitioners who provide nutrition support, counseling, and education to clients undergoing rehabilitation in inpatient/outpatient centers, group homes, transitional living centers, and industry.
Dietitians in Business and Communications (DBC) DPG	Professionals employed by, seeking employment in, or self-employed in the profit-making organizations of the food and nutrition industry.
Dietitians in General Clinical Practice DPG	Practitioners who possess a mosaic of professional skills, provide and/or manage nutrition care in settings ranging from acute care to long-term care, and maintain working knowledge in many clinical areas.
Dietitians in Nutrition Support (DNS) DPG	Practitioners integrating the science of enteral parenteral nutrition to provide appropriate nutrition support to individuals in inpatient and outpatient settings, including transplantation, home care, and pediatrics.
Food & Culinary Professionals DPG	Members who promote food education and culinary skills to enhance quality of life and health of the public.
Gerontological Nutritionists DPG	Practitioners who provide and manage nutrition programs and services to older adults in a variety of settings—community, home, health care facilities, and education and research facilities.

Table 2–1 continued

Dietetic Practice Group	Description
HIV/AIDS Dietetic Practice Group DPG	Dietetics professionals sharing cutting-edge information on nutrition management of HIV/AIDS and providing an avenue for research, monitoring, and advocacy for nutrition intervention.
Hunger and Environmental Nutrition DPG	Members who promote optimal nutrition and well-being for all people, now and in the future, acknowledging the interdependence of food and water security, health agriculture, and the environment.
Management in Food and Nutrition Systems DPG	Food and nutrition care managers generally employed in institutions, colleges, and universities; includes directors of departments of facilities, and administrative dietitians and technicians.
Nutrition Education for the Public (NEP) DPG	Practitioners involved in the design, implementation, and evaluation of nutrition education programs for target populations.
Nutrition Educators of Health Professionals (NEHP) DPG	Members involved in education and communication with physicians, nurses, dentists, and other health care professionals.
Nutrition Entrepreneurs (NE) DPG	Consultants in the business of developing and delivering nutrition-related services and/or products. Membership ranges from veteran business owners to members establishing new practices.
Nutrition in Complementary Care (NCC) DPG	Dietetics professionals interested in the study of alternative and complementary therapies.
Oncology Nutrition DPG	Nutrition professionals involved in the care of cancer patients, cancer prevention, and research.
Pediatric Nutrition DPG	Practitioners who provide nutrition services for the pediatric population in a wide variety of settings, including neonatal, nutrition support, and cystic fibrosis.
Public Health/Community Nutrition DPG	Nutrition professionals who provide nutrition services to all age groups in a community setting.
Renal Dietitians DPG	Practitioners who provide nutrition services to renal patients in dialysis facilities, clinics, hospitals, and private practice.
Research DPG	Members who conduct research in various areas of practice and are employed in the different practice settings of dietetics.
School Nutrition Services DPG	School food service directors and nutrition educators employed in child nutrition programs, and corporate dietitians working in companies supplying products or services to school food service operations.

(continues)

Table 2–1   continued

Dietetic Practice Group	Description
Sports, Cardiovascular and Wellness Nutritionists (SCAN) DPG	Nutrition professionals with expertise and skills in promoting the role of nutrition in physical performance, cardiovascular health, wellness, and disordered eating.
Vegetarian Nutrition DPG	Nutrition professionals in community, clinical, education, or food service settings who wish to learn about plant-based diets and provide support to individuals following vegetarian lifestyle.
Weight Management DPG	The Weight Management DPG supports the highest level of professional practice in the prevention and treatment of overweight and obesity throughout the life cycle.
Women's Health and Reproductive Nutrition DPG	Practitioners addressing women's nutrition care issues during preconception, pregnancy, postpartum, and lactation periods.

Source: ADA. "2003–2004 Dietetic Practice Groups." www.eatright.org/Public/ContinuingEducation/index_11383.cfm (accessed June 28, 2004).

balanced budget. DPGs offer networking opportunities with professionals with similar interests and provide significant opportunities for leadership responsibilities both within the DPG and the greater association.

Standards of Professional Practice

To evaluate the quality of dietetic services, the ADA appointed a task force in 1996 to review and update earlier standards to reflect the changing marketplace and to be more effective in helping members achieve their professional goals.[4,5] The standards were developed by a task force to assist the individual practitioner in systematically planning, implementing, evaluating, and adapting performance in every area of practice. The standards are broad statements that guide practice and are used by the DPGs to develop criteria by which their specific areas of practice can be evaluated. The six standards are the following:

1. Provision of services. Develops, implements, and promotes quality service based on client expectations and needs.
2. Application of research. Effectively applies, participates in, or generates research to enhance practice.
3. Communication and application of knowledge. Applies knowledge and communicates effectively with others.

4. Utilization and management of resources. Uses resources effectively and efficiently in practice.
5. Quality in practice. Systematically evaluates the quality and effectiveness of practice and revises practice as needed to incorporate the results of evaluation.
6. Continued competence and professional accountability. Engages in lifelong self-development to improve knowledge and skills that promote continued competence.

For further information about the rationale, indicators, and examples of outcomes of each of the standards, see Appendix C.

Position Papers

A position paper represents a consensus of viewpoints and professional interests and is used in many ways such as in media contacts, in drafting and testifying regarding legislation, and for communication with the public. A former president of the ADA described a position paper as: "a statement of the association's stance on an issue that affects the nutritional status of the public; it is derived from pertinent facts and data and is germane to the ADA's mission, vision, philosophy, and values."[6] Position papers are periodically updated or deleted and others added by the house of delegates.

The ADA has published approximately 40 position papers, and new ones are considered each year for adoption or for revision of existing papers.[7] The list of current papers is shown in Appendix D and copies are available from the ADA headquarters office. They may also be viewed from the ADA Web site: www.eatright.org/positions.html.[8]

Professional Code of Ethics

All professional groups adhere to a code of ethics that guides their practice. The ADA has followed a code since 1924 and the document has been revised and updated many times since the first one.[9] The code outlines 19 principles and includes procedures for the review process. The code is shown in Appendix A.

Salaries

The salary levels of dietitians and dietetic technicians have risen over the years, more in certain practice areas than others. These changes reflect both higher salaries due to the economy and also the increasingly important roles played by dietitians and dietetic technicians. In 1938 it was reported that the hospital dietitian earned a salary in the range of $1,080 to $7,000 per year. At that time, services such as room, board, and laundry were often supplied by the employer in addition to the salary. In positions other than hospitals, the salaries ranged from $1,200 to $4,000 per year. In 1946, the average salary was reported to be $3,000—not a significant improvement.[10]

In 1981, the ADA initiated the first survey of members that reported salaries along with other data regarding employment. At that time, the average yearly salary was reported to be $16,400 although the study did not equate all salaries with full-time practice and the actual salaries were probably higher.[11] The median yearly salary for dietitians in all areas of practice is shown in Table 2–2 for selected years 1993 through 2002.

Comparing salaries by areas of practice in dietetics, it is apparent that dietitians in consultation and business have the highest incomes (median of $60,000) while those earning the least ($42,825) are in clinical nutrition practice. Several factors account for differences in compensation levels including years in a position, educational level, job responsibilities, number of persons supervised, budget responsibility, and location.[12]

Table 2–2   Estimated Median Income for Registered Dietitians by Area of Practice (in dollars)

Practice Area	1993	1995	1997	1999	2002
Clinical	32,116	34,131	35,491	37,565	42,825
Food and Nutrition	40,441	43,964	44,924	48,924	55,000
Community Nutrition	31,810	33,902	34,870	37,990	43,200
Consultation/Business	40,365	43,374	46,040	48,810	60,000
Education/Research	39,427	42,764	45,211	47,040	54,800
All Areas	34,578	36,920	38,284	40,450	45,800

Source: Bryk, J.A. and T.K. Soto. Report on the 1993 Membership Database of the American Dietetic Association. *J Am Diet Assoc* 94(1994): 1433–1438.

Bryk, J.A. and T.H. Kornblum. Report on the 1995 Membership Database of the American Dietetic Association. *J Am Diet Assoc* 87(1997): 197–203.

Bryk, J.A. and T.K. Soto. Report on the 1997 Membership Database of the American Dietetic Association. *J Am Diet Assoc* 99(1999): 102–107.

Bryk, J.A. and T.K. Soto. Report on the 1999 Membership Database of the American Dietetic Association. *J Am Diet Assoc* 101(2001): 947–953.

Rogers, D. Report on the American Dietetic Association Dietetics Compensation and Benefits Survey. *J Am Diet Assoc* 103(2003): 243–255.

AFFILIATED UNITS OF THE AMERICAN DIETETIC ASSOCIATION

State and District Associations

Each of the 50 states and Puerto Rico are affiliates of the ADA and are organized with state and district associations. Membership in the ADA determines the membership in state affiliates because states generally charge no membership fees, and instead receive rebates from the ADA according to the number of members. A member of the ADA is automatically a member of a state affiliate.

The state organizations for the most part parallel the national organization. Each state elects its delegates to represent it in the HOD. The number of district organizations is determined by the states as well as how they fit into the state organization. The district groups provide educational and informational programs for the grassroots members. Most states have one or two meetings per year that provide continuing education opportunities for the members. Delegates from the state affiliates take state and/or member issues to the HOD for all members to have input into the functioning of the ADA.

American Dietetic Association Foundation

The foundation was established in 1966 as a means of providing monies for scholarships for prospective dietetic students and for members to continue their graduate education through fellowships. In the ensuing years, the foundation has experienced tremendous financial growth through its alignment with corporate sponsors and through ADA member campaigns. This additional financial growth has allowed the foundation to give increasing numbers of scholarships and to provide funding for significant research projects needed by the association and profession. A number of projects and services directly benefitted the public for several years through the National Center for Nutrition and Dietetics. Although the center no longer exists, the foundation continues to provide services for the public in various ways.

Washington Office

Since 1986, the association has staffed an office in Washington, D.C., in order to have a presence in the capital and to further the legislative efforts of the profession. This allows the association to be in touch with legislative issues as they are being considered and as they occur. Although these legislative and lobbying efforts required a tax status change for the association when first initiated, the benefits accrue to individual members directly and to consumers and the public indirectly.

The staff of the Washington office and ADA members work with legislators and government agencies to introduce and promote bills that further the interests of the profession and its members. Such a recent successful effort resulted in legislation allowing for third-party reimbursement to registered dietitians providing medical nutrition therapy in selected disease conditions.

SUMMARY

The ADA is the professional organization serving and promoting the interests of its members. The programs and initiatives administered by the association are for the benefit of the members and the public. The ADA is governed by elected and appointed volunteer members of boards, commissions, and committees, all of whom perform specific functions according to the bylaws of the ADA. Important as the functions are that the ADA provides for members, the association is recognized as the authoritative voice to the public with guidance regarding food and nutrition issues. The active promotion of policy that enhances the health and well-being of all individuals is accomplished through activities by members and by the Washington legislative office.

The mission statement "leading the future of dietetics" describes the overarching purpose of the ADA.

DEFINITIONS

Bylaws. Authoritative rules and regulations governing an association or group.

Chief Operating Officer. Person employed by the association to direct the headquarters office operations and implement the programs and fiscal affairs of the association. May also serve as an official spokesperson for the association on direction of the board of directors.

Governance. Activities involved in conducting the affairs of an organization.

House of Delegates. Body composed of members representing the membership who establish Standards, membership requirements, and other professional issues for the association.

Strategic Framework. Operational plans and strategies that shape the overall acivities and function of an organization.

REFERENCES

1. Fitz, P. The American Dietetic Association. *J Am Diet Assoc* 97(1997): 667–669.
2. ADA. "Strategic Plan 2003." www.eatright.org/member/governance (accessed 2/28/04).

3. See Note 2.

4. ADA. "Quality Assurance Committee: Standards of Practice: A Practitioner's Guide to Implementation." Chicago: The American Dietetic Association, 1986.

5. ADA. "The ADA Standards of Professional Practice for Dietetics Professionals." *J Am Diet Assoc* 98, no. 1(1998): 83–87.

6. Derelian, D. "President's Page: Positions—An Important Means of Fulfilling our Mission and Vision." *J Am Diet Assoc* 95(1995): 92.

7. ADA. "Position Paper Update for 2004." *J Am Diet Assoc* 104, no. 2(2004): 276–278.

8. ADA. "ADA Positions—The Voice of ADA." *Diet Pract* 2, no. 3(Winter 2002): 1.

9. ADA. "Code of Ethics for the Profession of Dietetics." *J Am Diet Assoc* 99, no. 1(1999): 109–113.

10. Cassell, J. *Carry the Flame: The History of the American Dietetic Association.* Chicago: The American Dietetic Association, 1990.

11. Baldyga, W.W. "Results from the 1981 Census of the American Dietetic Association." *J Am Diet Assoc* 83(1983): 343–348.

12. Rogers, D. "Report on the ADA 2002 Dietetics Compensation and Benefits Survey." *J Am Diet Assoc* 103, no. 2(2003): 243–255.

PART II

Education and Professional Development

CHAPTER 3

Educational Preparation in Dietetics

"As a profession, the one thing that we can predict is that the greatest change in our practice will be the change in knowledge and how we integrate new science into our daily practice."[1]

Outline

- Introduction
- Undergraduate Education
  - Current educational requirements
  - Eligibility requirements and accreditation standards
- Dietetic Education Programs
  - Didactic program in dietetics (DPD)
  - Coordinated program in dietetics (CP)
  - Dietetic technician (DT) program
- Trends in Dietetic Education
- Supervised Practice in Dietetics
- Education and Training of Dietetic Team Members
- Advanced-Level Education
  - Types of programs
  - Benefits of advanced study
  - The graduate experience
  - Research experience
- Summary

INTRODUCTION

Education is the key to dietetic practice and to the future of the profession. As with all professions, a specialized body of knowledge is required of individuals who practice in any area of dietetics. Because of the importance of education to the profession, the early leaders in dietetics set standards for education. The standards have been revised at intervals as the practice evolved and the needs of those being served also changed.

UNDERGRADUATE EDUCATION

The educational preparation of dietetics professionals begins in the undergraduate degree program. Study for the baccalaureate degree is based in the sciences, i.e., biological, physical, and social sciences and includes both a theoretical and applied course of study. The college or university offering a degree program plans a curriculum that meets both the educational standards of the American Dietetic Association (ADA) and the university requirements including courses for general education. A baccalaureate degree from an accredited college or university followed by an internship for supervised practice is required to complete all education requirements. Some programs offer the experience component concurrently with the degree as in the *coordinated program*. The curriculum that meets ADA educational standards is referred to as a *didactic program in dietetics (DPD)*. The dietetic technician (DT) similarly follows a course of study in a two-year college or institute that includes or is followed by supervised practice experience.

Current Educational Requirements

The model for dietetics practice (Figure 3–1) illustrates a fluid and flexible framework for practice in dietetics.[2] The core of the profession is food and nutrition services for individuals, groups, and communities. The dietetics professional provides services though communication and collaboration with others but also needs management, research, science, technology, and leadership to fully function.

The Commission on Accreditation for Dietetics Education (CADE) establishes the educational requirements and grants accreditation based on a self-study and a site visit to each college or university or other institution offering dietetics education.

A list of all programs, the "directory of programs," is available from a college or university department or from the ADA office.[3] The dietetics major is offered in at least one university in each state and in Hawaii and Puerto Rico.

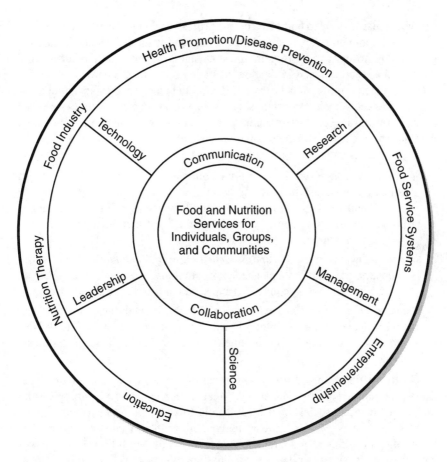

Figure 3–1 Model for Dietetics Practice. *Source:* Commission on Accreditation for Dietetics Education. *Accreditation Handbook.* Chicago: American Dietetic Association, 2002: p. 9.

Eligibility Requirements and Accreditation Standards

The ADA has set standards for dietetic education in various forms since 1924, but a major shift in requirements occurred when the Standards of Education were issued in 1987.[4] Prior to this time, a series of educational requirements delineated specific courses and competency-based minimum academic requirements.[5] The emphasis in the standards is on *outcomes* as opposed to earlier emphasis on the process involved in educating dietitians. The standards were revised and updated in 1997[6] and again in 2002.[7]

The standards apply to both didactic and professional practice programs and are based on a common body of knowledge, skills, and values. They encompass the goals and philosophy of a program, the students in the program, the curriculum, the program resources, and evaluation. In stating outcome standards for the education of dietetics professionals, there is flexibility in the way they are applied and evaluated because each institution is unique in terms of the programs offered and the resources available. Just as competencies represent the outcome of learning, the final product is a dietitian prepared for the first job.

The standards include the following:[8]

Standard One: Program Planning and Outcomes Assessment—The dietetics education program has clearly defined a mission, goals, program outcomes, and assessment measures and implements a systematic, continuous process to assess outcomes, evaluate goal achievement, and improve program effectiveness.

Standard Two: Curriculum and Student Learning Outcomes—The dietetics education program has a planned curriculum that provides for achievement of student learning outcomes and expected competence of the graduate.

Standard Three: Program Management—Management of the dietetics education program and availability of program resources are evident in defined processes and procedures and demonstrate accountability to students and the public.

The foundation *knowledge* and *skills* required in the didactic portion of educational programs are grouped under eight areas: communication, physiological and biological sciences, social sciences, research, food, nutrition, management, and health care systems. The same areas are required for the DT although the specific knowledge and skills differ. The knowledge and skills are followed by a list of *competencies* for the supervised practice portion of education.[9]

Each department or program providing dietetics education prepares a self-study document that describes how the standards are met in the program. This document, along with a site visit by registered dietitians (RDs) designated by ADA, is the basis for accreditation of the program. The purpose of the site visit is to assist the program in continual assessment that ensures qualified, competent graduates of the program. A program may be accredited for a period of 1 to 10 years. Yearly reports are submitted to ADA indicating that the program continues to provide education that meets the standards.

A schematic of dietitian and DT education is shown in Figure 3–2. Both the didactic and the experience portion of dietetics education are shown. Together, these result in competencies expected to be attained in order to perform in an entry-level position.

The CADE planners are guided by a model of lifelong learning showing the stages in professional growth (Figure 3–3). The model illustrates that professional

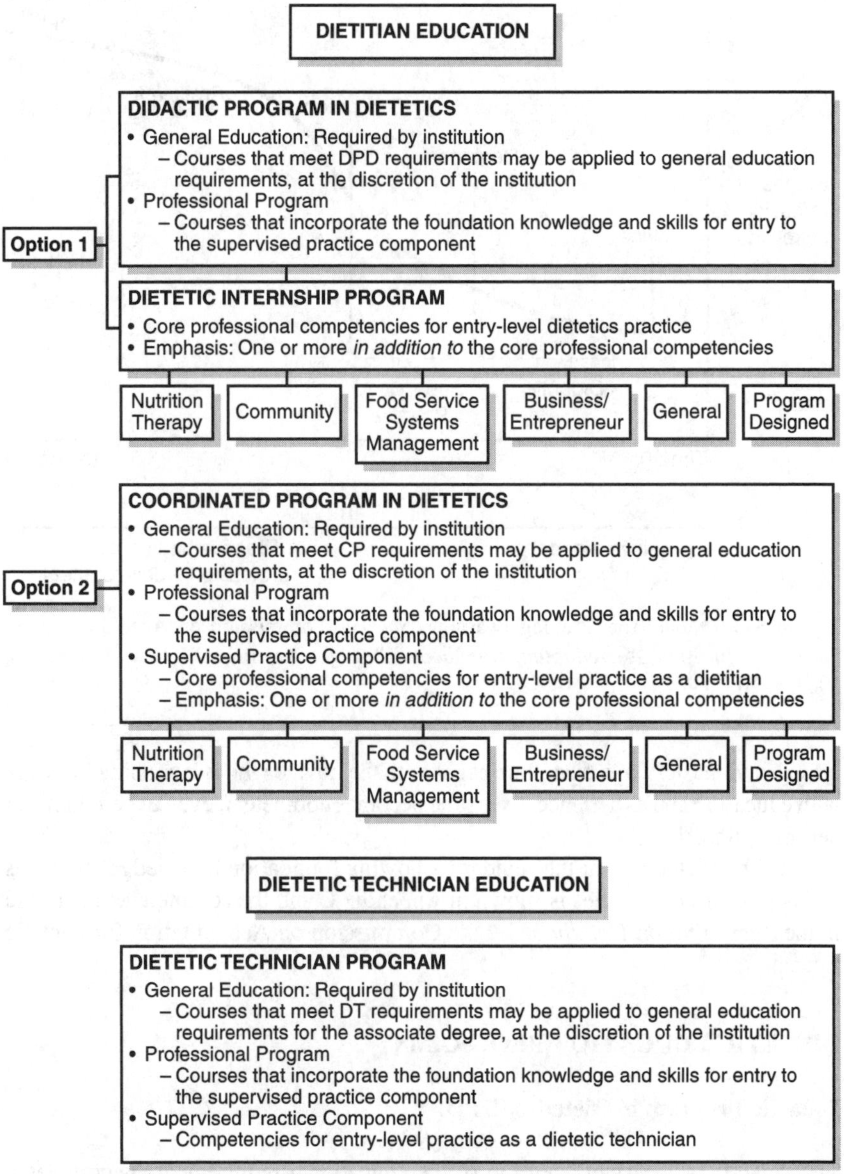

DIETITIAN EDUCATION

DIDACTIC PROGRAM IN DIETETICS
- General Education: Required by institution
  - Courses that meet DPD requirements may be applied to general education requirements, at the discretion of the institution
- Professional Program
  - Courses that incorporate the foundation knowledge and skills for entry to the supervised practice component

Option 1

DIETETIC INTERNSHIP PROGRAM
- Core professional competencies for entry-level dietetics practice
- Emphasis: One or more *in addition to* the core professional competencies

| Nutrition Therapy | Community | Food Service Systems Management | Business/ Entrepreneur | General | Program Designed |

COORDINATED PROGRAM IN DIETETICS
- General Education: Required by institution
  - Courses that meet CP requirements may be applied to general education requirements, at the discretion of the institution
- Professional Program
  - Courses that incorporate the foundation knowledge and skills for entry to the supervised practice component
- Supervised Practice Component
  - Core professional competencies for entry-level practice as a dietitian
  - Emphasis: One or more *in addition to* the core professional competencies

Option 2

| Nutrition Therapy | Community | Food Service Systems Management | Business/ Entrepreneur | General | Program Designed |

DIETETIC TECHNICIAN EDUCATION

DIETETIC TECHNICIAN PROGRAM
- General Education: Required by institution
  - Courses that meet DT requirements may be applied to general education requirements for the associate degree, at the discretion of the institution
- Professional Program
  - Courses that incorporate the foundation knowledge and skills for entry to the supervised practice component
- Supervised Practice Component
  - Competencies for entry-level practice as a dietetic technician

Figure 3–2 Schematic for Dietetics Education. *Source:* Commission on Accreditation for Dietetics Education. *Accreditation Handbook.* Chicago: American Dietetic Association, 2002: p. 1.

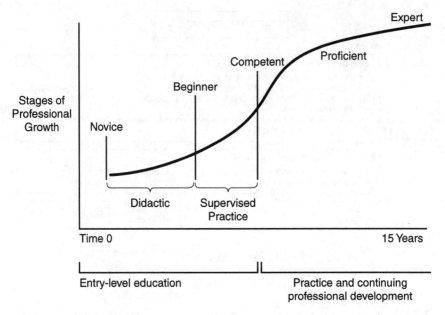

Figure 3–3   Model for Lifelong Learning. *Source:* Commission on Accreditation for Dietetics Education. *Accreditation Handbook.* Chicago: American Dietetic Association, 2002: p. 10.

growth and mastery of a discipline begin with the novice who is beginning but who, with education and experience, over time becomes competent, even expert, in his or her discipline.[10]

An abbreviated text of the standards showing foundation knowledge and skills and demonstrated abilities is shown in Appendix C and the complete text is found in the *Accreditation Handbook* by the Commission on Accreditation for Dietetic Education.[11]

DIETETIC EDUCATION PROGRAMS

Didactic Program in Dietetics (DPD)

The didactic or classwork portion of the educational requirements is completed during the degree program (either undergraduate or graduate). Following the degree, the student completes a supervised practice program. The traditional DPD is a 4-year undergraduate bachelor of science degree. In 2004, there were 229 accredited programs. Many of the courses required in the DPD are a combination of classroom and laboratory work, especially courses in food production, clinical nutrition, and in science courses such as chemistry and microbiology. During the latter part of the program, usually the senior year, the student applies to one or more dietetic internships through a computerized matching program. Notification is given in April or November about a "match" or acceptance to the student's program of choice.

Coordinated Program (CP)

In the CP, the didactic portion of a program plus supervised practice is completed during the course of study toward the degree. The student graduating from this program is thus prepared for entry-level practice upon completion of the degree. Currently, there are 50 CPs in the United States.

In most universities, students enter the CP for the junior and senior years. The programs are sometimes referred to as "two by two," meaning the first 2 years are general study and may be at a community or junior college and the last two include the integrated courses leading to the degree. Some programs may be longer than the traditional 4 years depending on the specific program requirements.

A university designates the criteria for admission to the CP. The selection criteria commonly include grade point average, writing skill, work experience, letters of recommendation, and sometimes, an interview. A minimum of 900 clock hours of supervised practice is required in the CP. The CP is intense in terms of time requirements and experiences but can lessen the time needed to prepare for practice. On completion of the degree, the graduate is eligible to take the registration examination.

Dietetic Technician (DT) Program

The DT program is similar to the coordinated program in that both didactic knowledge and skills and supervised practice are required in the program. The requirements are specified and programs are accredited by CADE. At present, there are 69 programs.[12] Graduates of the program are eligible to take the registration examination for DTs and for entry-level practice.

TRENDS IN DIETETIC EDUCATION

The education of the dietitian must be focused on the present and future practice roles the professionals are expected to fulfill. The traditional roles continue to expand as environmental, demographic, business, and health trends create new opportunities for practice. Several of these trends are identified by ADA as among those that are or will influence dietetic practice.[13]

These include:

- emphasis on outcomes and revenue
- demographics with more elderly among the population
- awareness of the relationship of diet to health
- governmental influence over health care
- technology and its increasing use
- emphasis on environmental issues
- vehicles for nutrition information
- the national economy with changing industries
- frequent restructuring of the health care industry
- consumer-driven economy
- rapidly changing food and nutrition knowledge base
- movement to a world economy
- changes in the education system and education resources

These trends have a number of implications for students in dietetics. One is that practitioners must be prepared by acquiring the knowledge and skills needed to function in regards to these trends and to anticipate that continuing education will be vital. Future-oriented continuing professional education is described as essential for keeping abreast of new developments, in anticipating change, and planning ahead.[14] The concept of multiskilling or cross-training has implications for educators as well as for students as they progress through an educational program.[15] This concept continues to gain attention because of predictions that cross-trained health professionals will be needed in health care, both to reduce health care costs and to develop a more efficient health care system. Skills such as leadership, communication skills, use of technology, ethical practice, counseling, marketing, and policy involvement are all part of dietetics training, and they also define the competent dietitian and DT.

The house of delegates (HOD) recently examined the influence of health care trends and health professions regulation, enrollment changes in higher education, and legal/ethical questions as among those issues affecting dietetic education.[16] The leadership team in the house has the responsibility of looking at future needs in the profession; in 2003, it developed a background paper about the outlook for dietetics education. As an outcome of discussion at the 2003 HOD annual meeting, a task force was appointed to create a new plan for the future of education and credentialing of the dietitian and DT.

SUPERVISED PRACTICE IN DIETETICS

Preprofessional or supervised practice is an essential step toward becoming an RD or registered dietitian technician (DTR). Supervised practice takes place in the work setting where students learn to apply their knowledge and skills under the direction and supervision of an RD preceptor. Successful completion of a supervised practice program establishes eligibility for an individual to write the registration examination and to apply for membership in the ADA. Competency in dietetics practice is the goal of supervised practice. *Competency* is regarded as the ability to carry out tasks within certain expected standards or parameters.

Supervised practice programs are based on the standards of education and the performance requirements for entry-level practice. All supervised programs are provided through an accredited program and must provide 450 hours (DTs) or 900 hours (dietitians) of experience. A current listing of all programs is available in *The Directory of Dietetics Programs* from the ADA.[17] The directory provides information about the length of the program, the number of students per class, estimated tuition, availability of financial aid, credit given toward an advanced degree, and the due date for the next accreditation. More detailed information may be obtained in the *Applicant Guide to Supervised Practice*.[18]

Although all supervised practice programs follows the same standards, there is flexibility in how the programs meet the standards. Although CADE accredits programs, it does not mandate the experiences or the amount of time in each area of practice. Each program sets the curriculum and experiences that meet the goals of the program and the needs of the student.

All programs plan the experiences around three key areas of activity in dietetics: clinical nutrition, food service management, and community dietetics. Programs that do not offer all the experiences in one institution will arrange with others in the community to provide the experiences.

The dietetic internship, the CP, and the DT program are the three types of supervised programs. The following questions are often asked when students apply for supervised practice programs:

What do students need to know before applying?　Students should know that a period of supervised experience is required to establish eligibility to become an RD or DT and that acceptance into a program is competitive. Further, the application process should begin early in the senior year in order to assemble all required materials and, if required by the program or desired by the student, to visit the program. Students applying for a dietetic internship will usually be required to participate in computer matching, and this information may be obtained from a program director or from the ADA office.

What are characteristics of successful applicants?　Generally, those with a 3.0 or above grade point average in food, nutrition, and management courses and better than average grades in biological and physical science courses will be considered first. Approximately 1 year of paid work experience or dietetics-related volunteer experience will increase the chances of being accepted.

What else is important to know?   In addition to good grades and having work experience, applicants are encouraged to investigate programs early to identify the specific admission criteria and apply to one or more programs. Successful applicants often apply to as many as three programs. If the program offers graduate credit during the supervised experience, the student will also need to apply to graduate school, and these admission dates will be important to note.

Applicants are encouraged to be flexible and willing to relocate.

EDUCATION AND TRAINING OF DIETETIC TEAM MEMBERS

Through role delineation studies conducted by the ADA in the 1980s, the roles and responsibilities of dietetic team members were identified. The comprehensive studies described the work of dietitians in three areas of practice: clinical dietetics, food service management, and community dietetics.[19] A second role delineation study included DTs and clearly pointed out the differences in the roles of both groups. A comparison of the characteristics of the dietetics team is shown in Table 3–1.

In 1995, the Commission on Dietetic Registration updated earlier studies in a practice audit.[20] Generally, the results from the 1995 audit confirmed those from the earlier role delineation study.

ADVANCED-LEVEL EDUCATION

Advanced-level education may be described as continuing or postprofessional education as well as graduate education. More baccalaureate students are pursuing graduate degrees; more employers are requiring advanced degrees or training; and more disciplines are becoming specialized, thus requiring advanced level education. Continuing education is discussed in greater detail in Chapter 5. Graduate education is formal study beyond a baccalaureate degree that leads to an advanced degree, usually the masters or doctoral degree. Graduate study involves concentrated study in a specific academic area.

Among the important purposes of advanced education are opportunities for individuals to explore new ideas and gain a higher level of knowledge and understanding required to recognize and fully discharge personal, social, and professional responsibilities.[21] Practical benefits also accrue, including the possibility of career advancement and financial gains.

Table 3-1 Comparison of Characteristics of Professional Members of the Dietetic Team

	Dietary Managers	Dietetic Technicians	Dietitians
Education/Training	Postsecondary education program approved by Dietary Managers Association (DMA) (site-based or independent study*) for those employed in food service positions: 120 clock hours of classroom instruction 150 clock hours of supervised field experience	2-year community college programs, approved by ADA (site-based or independent study) for full- or part-time students who may or may not be employed in food service positions: Associate degree (ADA-approved) including 450 clock hours of supervised field experience or Graduates of BS degree/ADA-approved didactic program in dietetics who add the supervised field experience component from an ADA-approved dietetic technician program	4-year baccalaureate degree from an ADA-approved *didactic program in dietetics* consisting of: Baccalaureate degree (ADA approved) and ADA-accredited supervised preprofessional experience (at least 900 clock hours), usually administered through a different institution or 4-year baccalaureate degree from an ADA-accredited *coordinated program in dietetics* consisting of: Baccalaureate degree including 900 hours of supervised preprofessional experience administered through the degree-granting institution

(continues)

47

Table 3–1 continued

	Dietary Managers	Dietetic Technicians	Dietitians
Degree Attained	None; although some dietary managers could have earned degrees previously from 2- or 4-year colleges. One route to eligibility to take the certified dietary manager (CDM) examination is to have a BS degree in nutrition	Associate degree (graduates of a 2-year ADA-approved dietetic technician program) Baccalaureate degree (graduates of a 4-year ADA-approved didactic program in dietetics)	Baccalaureate degree Masters degree (in some universities the coordinated programs and the supervised preprofessional experience programs are at the graduate-degree level)
Credential	CDM National examination administered by the Certifying Board of Dietary Managers	DTR National examination administered by the Commission on Dietetic Registration (CDR)	RD national examination administered by the CDR
Professional Organization	DMA One Pierce Place, Suite 1220W Itasca, IL 60143-1277	The ADA 216 West Jackson Boulevard Chicago, IL 60606-6995	The ADA 216 West Jackson Boulevard Chicago, IL 60606-6995
Primary Employment Opportunities	Long-term care facilities Life-care centers Hospitals Schools Correctional facilities	Hospitals Long-term care facilities Community nutrition programs	Hospitals Long-term care facilities Community nutrition programs Corporations (e.g., pharmaceutical, food manufacturers, food distributors, contract management) Self-employment

Table 3–1 continued

	Dietary Managers	Dietetic Technicians	Dietitians
Type of Work	Manages/supervises food service operations	Supervises/provides patient/ client nutrition services Supervises/manages food service operations Provides nutrition education	Manages/provides patient/client nutrition services Manages food service operations Develops/provides nutrition education programs Manages dietetic consulting services

*These programs are also called *correspondence* or *distance learning.*
Source: Kane, M.T., C.A. Estes, D.A. Colton, and C.S. Eltoft. "Role Delineation for Dietetics Practitioners: Empirical Results." *J Am Diet Assoc* 90(1990): 1124–1133.

Types of Programs

The master of science (MS) degree usually requires 1 to 2 years of full-time study and may be longer depending on the major area of study, the research undertaken, and whether the student is employed while working toward the degree. In some universities, the MS will be offered with the option of a thesis or a creative component entailing either extra course work or a project.

The doctor of philosophy (PhD) degree requires at least 3 to 5 years of full-time study. The PhD or the EdD (Doctor of Education) may be offered. Original research is required for either degree, the type depending on the field of study. The doctoral degree is considered the "terminal degree," although it may be followed by post-doctoral academic work.

In some professions, a professional degree may be awarded at either the masters or doctoral level. This degree will generally have a title descriptive of the profession (i.e., MD for medical practice, JD for law, DDS for dental practice, and MBA for business administration).

Benefits of Advanced Study

Although an advanced degree is not required to take the registration examination in dietetics, there are valid reasons why dietitians pursue advanced study. In the 2002 Dietetics Compensation and Benefits Survey,[22] it was reported that 48 percent of RDs hold a master's or doctoral degree. Of DTRs, 23 percent have a BS degree and 3 percent a masters degree.

The benefits of an advanced degree include the development of intellectual skills, including the ability to master complex information, to problem solve, and to explore new ideas. Career benefits include the development of advanced practice skills, the in-depth exploration of subjects in one's area of practice, and the acquisition of new perspectives.[23] Career advancement and preparation for a career change are often reasons dietitians pursue graduate study. Dietitians who are prepared to perform in multiskilled or cross-trained positions will usually rely on graduate education to increase both knowledge and practice skills. The types of positions dietitians assume as they progress up the career ladder are usually those with increasing responsibility and autonomy, and they require managerial and leadership skills. In addition, competition for jobs may increase the demand for an advanced degree. New and expanding career options, and the job market in general, affect demand and availability of persons prepared to enter the new job markets and, in turn, influence dietitians in their education choices. Graduate education provides an opportunity to develop expertise that allows them to assume leadership roles.

The financial advantages of an advanced degree in dietetics are demonstrated in Figure 3–4.[24] Attaining a masters degree increases the hourly wages of dietitians

RD hourly wage by education level

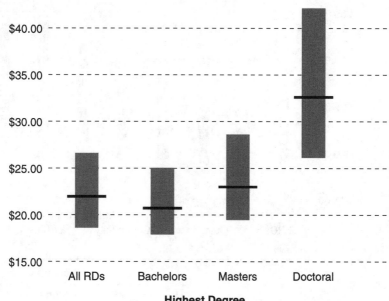

Highest Degree

	No.	Percentiles		
		25th	**50th**	**75th**
All RDs	8.621	$18.75	$22.00	$26.79
Doctoral degree	272	$26.04	$32.57	$42.06
Masters degree	3,823	$19.39	$23.13	$28.57
Bachelors degree	4,497	$17.92	$20.83	$25.00

Figure 3–4   Rogers, D. "Report on the ADA 2002 Dietetics Compensation and Benefits Survey." *J Am Diet Assoc* 103, no. 2 (2003): p. 248.

by $2.30 and the doctoral degree by $11.74. On an annualized basis, the difference in salary between a bachelors degree and a doctoral degree is $24,420. For DTRs, the hourly wage difference between an associate and a masters degree is $6.83 or $14,206 per year. State licensure and specialty certification also affect salaries, again often equated with advanced study. Dietitians working in practice areas that often require advanced degree, i.e., food and nutrition management, consultation and business, and education and research, earn the highest salaries (Figure 3–5).

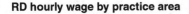

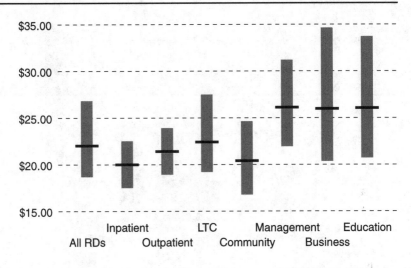

			Percentiles	
	No.	25th	50th	75th
All RDs	8,621	$18.75	$22.00	$26.79
Acute care/inpatient	2,420	$17.55	$19.95	$22.62
Ambulatory care	1,180	$18.99	$21.39	$24.07
Long-term care	1,020	$19.23	$22.61	$27.55
Community	981	$16.83	$20.51	$24.73
Food and nutrition management	1,198	$22.00	$26.22	$31.26
Consultation and business	924	$20.43	$26.04	$34.62
Education and research	539	$20.77	$26.17	$33.65

Figure 3–5 RD Hourly Wage by Practice Area. *Source:* Rogers, D. "Report on the ADA 2002 Dietetics Compensation and Benefits Survey." *J Am Diet Assoc* 103, no. 2 (2003): p. 249.

A further justification for the RD to pursue graduate study is for continuing education credit to maintain registration status. State licensure regulations often mandate an advanced degree as well.

Active membership in the ADA is available to an individual holding a masters or doctoral degree in one of the following areas: dietetics, food and nutrition, food science, or food service systems management. The degree must be from a regionally accredited college or university.

Gaining research skills and understanding research articles and reports is a further benefit of graduate study. All dietitians apply research in their practice and need to demonstrate the ability to interpret current research and basic statistics. However, designing and participating in more formal research usually occurs at the graduate level.

The Graduate Experience

Information about graduate programs offering degrees related to dietetics, their location, emphasis areas, and a contact person is available in the *ADA Directory of Programs* and on the Internet.[25] Many other universities also offer graduate degrees and may be contacted. Prospective students will find it helpful to talk with faculty and to request college catalogs and departmental information before applying. No two programs are alike, and the best fit between the student and a program will be important once the student is admitted to the program. Universities that give students an active role in departmental activities and who give individual time and attention in a mentoring and supportive atmosphere will greatly enhance the graduate experience. The faculty, the departmental research, and the availability of financial aid through graduate assistantships should also be explored. Assistantships not only provide financial aid but give the student teaching, research, and administrative experience according to assignments.

Research Experience

The selection of a research study by the student with the advisor is based on the area of interest, the need as determined by a literature search, and the feasibility (cost, time involvement, availability of equipment and/or subjects). Ongoing departmental faculty research can provide a way for the student to assume a part of the research for his or her thesis.

The process of investigating a problem, reviewing the literature to support the need for the study, planning and implementing the study, collecting and analyzing data, and writing a clear and well-developed document that is accepted by a graduate faculty committee is a significant effort. The research experience involves initiative, critical thinking, problem solving, and ethics. These are aspects of professional function that are vital to success in life, as well as a career. The successful completion of a research study often launches a student into publishing the results and into further research, thus making an important contribution to scholarship as well.

SUMMARY

Dietetics education has evolved over time but has always been based on preparing the student for professional practice. The ADA designates the educational standards that are followed by all dietetics programs, thus ensuring competent practitioners. With a background of academic knowledge and practical skills, dietitians and DTs are prepared for a wide variety of careers as described in other chapters in this book.

Almost half of practicing dietitians today hold or are working toward a graduate or advanced degree. There are benefits in doing so, among them the attainment of research competence, continuing education for personal and professional growth, and career enhancement. If the trend continues, ever-larger numbers of dietitians will seek an advanced degree and will thereby bring expertise to bear on practical problems. The outcome will be a healthy and informed public and heightened recognition of the dietitian as the expert in food and nutrition.

DEFINITIONS

Accreditation. Process whereby a private nongovernmental agency or association grants public recognition to an institution that meets the necessary qualifications and periodic evaluations. In dietetics, the process includes a self-study by the institution and a site visit.

Basic Requirement. Fundamental requirements for dietetics education programs.

Communications Technology. Electronic and automatic working channels that lead to interaction between the source and the receiver.

Competency-Based Education. Learning that is functionally adequate in performing the tasks and assuming the role of a specified position.

Coordinated Program. A degree program combining didactic and experiential learning.

Cross-Training. Process of learning how to perform in two or more occupations.

Didactic Instruction. Knowledge acquired through classroom instruction.

Dissertation. A paper reporting original research required for the doctoral degree.

Experiential Learning. Learning attained through actual experiences.

Multiskilling. Process of becoming proficient in more than one procedure or skill.

Preceptor. Person who guides, mentors, and evaluates a student during the supervised practice experience.

Preprofessional Practice. Experiences in real-life situations prior to an entry-level position.

Self-Assessment. Self-examination of one's status or needs.

Supervised Practice. Learning experiences associated with activities in selected situations that enable the student to apply knowledge, develop and retain skills, and develop professionally.

REFERENCES

1. Parks, S.C., M.R. Schiller, and J. Bryk. "President's Page: Investment in Our Future— The Role of Science and Scholarship in Developing Knowledge for Dietetics Practice." *J Am Diet Assoc* 94(1994): 1159–1161.

2. Commission on Accreditation for Dietetics Education. *Accreditation Handbook.* Chicago: American Dietetic Association, 2002.

3. *Directory of Dietetic Programs.* American Dietetic Association, 2003–2004.

4. Bruening K., B.E. Mitchell, and M.M. Pfeiffer. "2002 Accreditation Standards for Dietetic Education." *J Am Diet Assoc* 102, no. 4(2002): 566–577.

5. Wenberg, B. "Dietetics Education: Past, Present, and Future." In *Proceedings of Future Search Conference Challenging the Future of Dietetic Education and Credentialing— Dialogue, Discovery, and Directions.* Chicago: The American Dietetic Association and Commission on Registration, 1994, pp. 3–12.

6. Gilmore, G.A., J.O. Maillet, and B.E. Mitchell. "Determining Educational Preparation Based on Job Competencies of Entry-Level Dietetics Practitioners." *J Am Diet Assoc* 97(1997): 306–316.

7. See Note 4.

8. Ibid.

9. See Note 2.

10. See Note 4.

11. See Note 2.

12. White, J. Personal Communicating. American Dietetic Association. Chicago: April 2004.

13. "Nutrition Leadership." *ADA Cour* 34, no. 11(1995): 4–8.

14. Berenbaum, S. "Future-Oriented Continuing Professional Education." *Topics in Clinical Nutrition* 10(1995): 66–70.

15. Sandoval, W.M. "Multiskilling and Dietetics Education." *DEP Line* 142(1996): 5–8.

16. HOD Backgrounder. *Dietetics Education and the Needs for the Future.* www.eatright.org/membr/85_17558.cfm (accessed April 1, 2004).

17. See Note 3.

18. *Applicant Guide to Supervised Practice,* American Dietetic Association. Chicago: 2003–2004.

19. Kane, M.T., C.A. Estes, D.A. Colton, and C.S. Eltoft. "Role Delineation for Dietetics Practitioners: Empirical Results." *J Am Diet Assoc* 90(1990): 1124–1133.

20. Kane, M.T., A.S. Cohen, E.R. Smith, C. Lewis, and C. Reidy. "1995 Commission on Dietetic Registration Dietetics; Practice Audit. *J Am Diet Assoc* 96(1996): 1292–1301.

21. Brooks, P. "Point of View. Graduate Learning as Apprenticeship." Abstract. *Chronicle of Higher Education* XLIII(1996): A52.

22. Rogers, D. "Report on the ADA 2002 Dietetics Compensation and Benefits Survey." *J Am Diet Assoc* 103, no. 2(2003): 342–355.

23. Gaffney, N.A. *Graduate School and You: A Guide for Prospective Graduate Students,* 4th ed. Washington DC: Council on Graduate Schools, 1996.

24. See Note 3.

CHAPTER 4

Credentialing of Dietetic Practitioners

"Experts at curing diseases are inferior to specialists who warn against disease. Experts in the use of medicines are inferior to those who recommend proper diet."[1]

Outline

- Introduction
- Development of Certification and Registration
- Commission on Dietetic Registration
- Specialty Certification
- Licensure of Dietitians
- Summary

INTRODUCTION

The term *dietitian* was one that evolved over time. Early practitioners were called dietologists, dietists, and dietotherapists. Before the American Dietetic Association (ADA) was formed, a dietitian was described as "a person who specializes in the knowledge of food and can meet the demands of the medical profession for diet therapy" and this adequately described the professional for many decades.[2]

The developing science of food and nutrition formed the basis for the organization of a group of practicing professionals. One of the earliest concerns of this group was the overwhelming amount of food faddism and fallacies between the general public and other professionals. It was difficult, if not impossible, for the public to determine who was a credible source of information and to separate fact

57

from fiction between the many medical and health claims for specific foods and procedures.

This early concern for protection of the public by disseminating the knowledge of dietitians has continued to the present time. Not only did it lead to the national organization of dietitians who could promote the professionals as having expertise in "diet-therapy, teaching, social welfare, and administration," but it served as the impetus to begin thinking about credentialing of practitioners.[3]

Another concern came forward at the second annual meeting of the ADA in 1918 and that was the "need to distinguish between dietitians with a college degree and special training in some scientific work and the ones with lesser training."[4]

This was perhaps the first formal reference to credentialing. The 1926 president of the association, Florence Smith, urged that the group should establish the standards for dietitians and that state or national registration could be the answer. In 1929, a study of national registration was initiated and the following definition of a dietitian was adopted: "Any person who is qualified for membership in The American Dietetic Association is by virtue of uniform basic training and required experience, entitled to be designated as a dietitian."[5] In the 1950s the association appointed a committee to formally study state licensing of dietitians. The issue of *specialties* in practice also surfaced with the suggestion that membership should be expanded to include others who were well-qualified in the many specialties embraced within the definition of dietetics.[6] However, it was in the late 1950s that educational and membership requirements were varied to accommodate practitioners with similar basic preparation but in specialized areas of practice.

A generalist (defined as a dietitian who could perform in all areas of practice, e.g., a single dietitian in a small hospital or as one who could move from one practice area to another) versus the specialist (a dietitian wanting to restrict his or her practice in one area, i.e., clinical or food service) surfaced and was thoroughly debated. The generalist role was advanced by the following themes:

1. All dietitians are the same.
2. Dietitians can move from one area of practice (food service to public health for example) to another without additional training.
3. Greater external recognition of the term *dietitian* was established.

By contrast, the specialized role was driven by the following themes:

1. The explosion of knowledge and technology requiring each dietitian to know more and more about less and less.
2. The need to differentiate among dietitians with varying skills and knowledge, advanced education, and experience gained on the job.
3. The emergence of part-time employment opportunities.
4. New, innovative practice areas (school food service, consultant to nursing home, enteral and parenteral nutrition techniques, and nutrition support).

DEVELOPMENT OF CERTIFICATION
AND REGISTRATION

In the 1960s, a committee was established to study licensure, registration, and certification. Registration was the process chosen at that time by the house of delegates and membership and an amendment to the constitution was approved for the "Final Revised Proposal for Professional Registration" in 1969. A committee then began the implementation process of putting a registration of members into effect. A detailed account of the implementation and a review of the first 5 years of professional registration was published in the *Journal of the American Dietetic Association* in 1974.[7]

The professional registration system adopted by the association differed significantly from other health professional certification systems at that time in that candidates had to pass a national examination, and registered dietitians (RDs) had to document evidence of continuing education in each 5-year period to renew registration. Thus registration was designed as a voluntary process ensuring competency of dietitians through the qualifications required to take the examination for registration, passing the examination, and formal continuing education. All this was evidence of the concern of the profession for the health, safety, and welfare of the public by encouraging high standards of performance by dietetic practitioners as stated in the amendment to the constitution.[8]

Ninety-three percent of the membership was registered by the end of the 1970s with the majority "grandfathered" in during the period before establishment of the examination.

COMMISSION ON DIETETIC REGISTRATION

The Commission on Dietetic Registration (CDR) is the agency responsible for maintaining the registration process for the ADA. This group develops the examination for registration and sets the standards for certification, recertification, and the code of ethics and issues credentials to individuals who meet these standards.[9] The examination is now administered online (prior to this it was offered in written form at designated sites twice a year) and is available whenever an applicant chooses. The examination is also available in other countries with which the ADA has reciprocity. The process by which the 75 clock hours of continuing education are accumulated is also determined by the CDR, which specifies the educational activities that qualify.

In 2001, the CDR implemented a new process for continued certification termed the *Professional Development Portfolio* (PDP).[10] By this plan, the individual assumes the responsibility for learning, professional development, and career direction. The PDP requires each practitioner to first engage in self-reflection, followed by assessment and goal setting. This is followed by the development of a 5-year plan that reflects a critical analysis of goals and the steps to be taken to maintain professional competency. After a pilot study from 1998 to 2000, the new procedure was initiated in 2001 with 6,000 dietitians submitting their learning plan.[11,12]

The eligibility requirements for dietitians to take the registration examination are the following:[13]

1. Education. Minimum of a baccalaureate degree from an accredited college or university and completion of the current Standards of Education as approved by the ADA.
2. Supervised practice. To be met in an accredited dietetic internship or accredited coordinated program.

Dietetic technicians wishing to take the registration examination must meet the following eligibility requirements:

1. Education. An associate or baccalaureate degree from an accredited college or university and completion of approved courses in an ADA-approved dietetic technician program or a didactic program in dietetics.
2. Supervised practice. Completion of supervised field experience as stipulated in an ADA-approved dietetic technician program.

To remain registered, an RD is required to pay yearly dues and engage in 75 clock hours of continuing education for recertification. A registered dietetic technician pays dues and must accrue 50 clock hours for recertification.

SPECIALTY CERTIFICATION

In 1986, the concept of *specialized practice* was approved by the house of delegates. The ADA defined a *specialty* as an advanced level of practice that responds to a defined area of need and requires demonstrated competence exceeding that for entry level. Specialty areas must have a substantial and verifiable knowledge base, an identified dimension of advanced practice, and a reasonable pool of practitioners. Three areas of practice were selected: pediatric nutrition, renal nutrition, and metabolic nutrition care.[14] The first members were chartered in 1994. The metabolic nutrition care specialty was later discontinued.[15] Specialists were given the credential: board-certified specialist in pediatric, renal, or metabolic care.

A further area of recognition was developed in 1993[16] for those practicing at advanced levels in any area of dietetics. The "Fellow of the ADA" was available until 2003 for those having an advanced degree, 8 years of practice, plus other documented professional achievements. This recognition was discontinued because of limited participation of members of the association.

LICENSURE OF DIETITIANS

Licensing of professionals occurs through legislative action in each state. It is a separate process from registration, which is a national credential. Licensure provisions differ somewhat from state to state, but essentially the process protects the title *dietitian* and, depending on the legislation, may also protect the scope of practice in dietetics by ensuring that only qualified professionals may practice in a state. Most states that have passed licensure legislation (currently 33) use the RD eligibility requirements in determining licensure eligibility.

The ADA provides assistance to states by publishing the document: "Licensure/ Entitlement for Dietitians" with definitions, terminology, and titles, plus a model scope of practice and sample bills (see the ADA Web site: http://www. eatright.org.).

SUMMARY

Dietitians continue to desire recognition and differentiation among their peers that is visible and can be communicated to other professional practitioners. The credentialing program does this. The RD has become valued to the point that most individuals consider it synonymous with dietitian. Employers view it as a mandatory credential to practice. Credentials have also been used in international markets and jobs to describe individuals and job qualifications. For dietitians and technicians, this is a plus as the world moves toward a global practice and global economy.

Consumers will always demand credentials of some kind. As consumers recognize that the credentials of the ADA provide assurance that the practitioners are competent and can provide services they want, the demand will continue to rise. More significantly, these credentials will enhance the RD's efforts to describe the diversity and to obtain a competitive advantage in the practice of dietetics in the United States and internationally.

DEFINITIONS

Certification. The process by which a nongovernmental agency or association grants recognition to an individual who has met certain predetermined qualifications specified by that agency or association (e.g., registration for dietitians and dietetic technicians administered by the CDR).

Credentialing. Formal recognition of professional or technical competence as by certification or licensure.

Licensure. Process by which an agency of government grants permission to an individual to engage in a given occupation on finding that the applicant has attained the minimal degree of competency necessary to ensure that the public health, safety, and welfare are reasonably well-protected.

Practitioner. One who practices in a profession or occupation.

Registration. (*See* Credentialing.)

Scope of Practice. Extent of or dimensions of activities performed in an area of practice.

REFERENCES

1. Needham, J. *Clerks and Craftsmen in China and the West. Lectures and Addresses on the History of the Science and Technology.* Cambridge, MA: University Press, 1970.

2. Cassell, J. *Carry the Flame: The History of the American Dietetic Association.* Chicago: The American Dietetic Association, 1990.

3. Ibid.

4. Ibid.

5. Ibid.

6. Perry, E. "Report of the Executive Board." *J Am Diet Assoc* 26(1950): 949–957.

7. Bogle, M.L. "Registration: The *Sine Qua Non* of a Competent Dietitian." *J Am Diet Assoc* 64(1974): 616–620.

8. ADA. *Constitution of the American Dietetic Association, as Amended.* Chicago: The American Dietetic Association, 1971.

9. ADA. "Bylaws of American Dietetic Association." Revised March 10, 2002. www.eatright.org/member/governance/85_12428.cfm (accessed March 1, 2004).

10. Weddle, D.O., S.P. Himsburg, N. Collins, and R. Lewis. "The Professional Development Portfolio Process: Setting Goals for Credentialing." *J Am Diet Assoc* 102, no. 10(2002): 1439–1444.

11. Ibid.

12. Keim, K.S., G.E. Gates, and C.A. Johnson. "Dietetics Professionals Have a Positive Perception of Professional Development." *J Am Diet Assoc* 101, no. 7(2001): 820–824.

13. Keim, K.S., C.A. Johnson, and G.E. Gates. "Learning Needs and Continuing Professional Education Activities of Professional Development Portfolio Participants." *J Am Diet Assoc* 101, no. 6(2001): 697–702.

14. ADA. *Directory of Dietetics Programs, 1977–1998.* Chicago: The American Dietetic Association, 1997.

15. Bogle, M.L., L. Balogun, J. Cassell, A. Catakis, H.J. Holler, and C. Flynn. "Achieving Excellence in Dietetic Practice: Certification of Specialists and Advanced-Level Practitioners." *J Am Diet Assoc* 93(1993): 149–150.

16. Personal communication with C. Reidy of the ADA, January 20, 2004.

CHAPTER 5

The Dietetics Professional

"Ethics in dietetics practice: Complicated issues for a complicated time."[1]

Outline

- Introduction
- Ethical Practice
- Political Awareness
  — ADA priorities
- Lifelong Professional Development
  — Lifelong learning
  — Delivery of learning
  — Self-responsibility for learning
- Legal Basis of Practice
  — Regulations affecting dietitians
  — Regulations affecting practice
- Evidence-Based Practice
- Summary

INTRODUCTION

Professional practice can be defined in several ways, first and foremost, as practice based on specialized learning and training and adherence to a code of ethical actions adopted by the group. Dietitians who develop a professional portfolio for registration status are familiar with the process involved, such as a plan for continued competence in practice with supporting goals and measures to reach the goals. The emphasis is on continued learning and self-monitoring, both distinguishing features of a professional.

Professional standards of practice have been developed for the dietetics profession as a whole and specific standards in several areas of practice (see Appendix C).[2] The standards define desirable and achievable levels of performance. They are statements of the dietetic professional's responsibility for providing services in all areas of practice and describe the minimum levels of performance expected. The benefits of having standards that apply to all are shown in the following ways:

- They provide a guide to the knowledge, skills, judgments, and attitudes that are needed in dietetics practice.
- They represent performance criteria against which all dietetics professionals may be compared by consumers, employers, and colleagues.
- They provide direction for the development of dietetics services.
- They encourage research to validate dietetics practice, services, and effectiveness.
- They generate data to lead to improved delivery of dietetics services.

In addition to becoming proficient in an area of practice and continually monitoring performance, there are related areas of knowledge and practice that support and enhance competence but are usually not evident in a job description. Specifically, the areas to be discussed in this chapter include ethical practice, political awareness, lifelong professional development, the legal bases of practice, and evidence-based practice.

ETHICAL PRACTICE

The Professional Code of Ethics[3] is the guiding document for ethical practice in dietetics. The framework in which such policies are developed is the hallmark of an effective value structure that includes the following:[4]

- Guiding values and commitments make sense and are clearly communicated.
- Organizational leaders are personally committed, credible, and willing to take action on the values they espouse.
- Values are integrated into the normal channels of management decision making and are reflected in the organization's critical activities.
- The organization's systems and structures support and enforce its values.
- Managers throughout the organization have the decision-making skill, knowledge, and competencies needed to make ethically sound decisions on a day-to-day basis.

In practice, many situations arise in which it is not always clear what the course of action should be to be considered ethical. Ethical conflicts of interest and poor business practices are examples of how ethical conduct impacts dietetic practice.[5–7] Besides conflicts of interest, issues of confidentiality, promotion and endorsement of products, and recognition of professional judgment may be faced at times.

In clinical practice, activities related to dispensing supplementation advice and conducting online counseling and consultation can lead to liability risks, making it important to be familiar with laws and regulations as well as the code of ethics.[8] Other instances in which ethical conduct must be considered are disclosure of confidential information, accepting gifts, discussing patients, charting, or giving information about prices or salaries. In such cases, open discussion with trusted peers or a supervisor before action is the best course to follow. A personal code of conduct that espouses integrity, fairness, and a sense of always wanting to do "the right thing" helps make difficult decisions about ethical questions easier. The manager/ leader assists in developing organization practices and policies that promote ethical practice. Such policies include purchasing, financial management, patient care issues, and information provided patients and clients among others—and, the manager/leader sets an example for ethical behavior built on openness and trust.

Ethical and legal issues in nutrition, hydration, and feeding are discussed in an ADA position paper along with guidelines for nutrition and hydration of persons through the life span. An ethical deliberation process is shown in Table 5–1.[9]

Several resources available for ethical dilemmas in dietetics are discussed by Holler.[10]

POLITICAL AWARENESS

Dietitians in all areas of practice are influenced by actions of governmental bodies because the accreditation of programs and credentialing of professionals has the backing and authority of a governmental agency or group. For example, state licensure must be enacted by a state legislative action. Congress and state legislatures enact laws regarding health care: the type, the reimbursement for those working in health care, and the qualifications of practitioners. The Food and Drug Administration regulates the safety of drugs and foods and therefore what is allowed on the market. Similarly, the U.S. Department of Agriculture (USDA) regulates meat and poultry products on the market. The USDA issues dietary guidance such as the Food Pyramid and, with the Department of Health and Human Services, the Dietary Guidelines. The USDA also issues regulations pertaining to school nutrition programs; the women's, infants and children's programs; and the food stamp program. The National Academy of Sciences publishes nutrient intake guides for the population. Other agencies issue guidelines for staffing and procedures in all health care institutions receiving federal or state monies.

ADA Priorities

The ADA has been involved in public policy since the 1960s and in 1980 established an office in Washington, D.C., with staff who perform lobbying activities,

Table 5–1   Suggested Ethical Deliberative Process

1. Clarify the moral question—the first statement of the moral problem.
2. Recreate the context.
   a. gather data
   b. relevant facts
   c. relevant values
3. Name stakeholders and their relationships.
4. Identify ways of ethical thinking used by the stakeholders.
   a. rules thinking—ethics is about doing what is right by following the rules
   b. roles thinking—ethics is about being true to yourself and following your sense of virtue
   c. goals thinking—ethic is about producing good outcomes regardless of the rules and virtues
5. Determine practical limits to the situation: policies, laws, standards, and codes.
6. Center on balancing the patient's known beliefs and preferences with the best interests of the patient.
7. Respect advance directives.
8. Assume the patient has decisional capacity.
9. If decisional capacity is in question, determine decisional incapacity and select substitute decision maker if necessary.
10. Restate the ethical problem.
11. Search for possible options.
12. Test the various options.
    a. check through each option for:
       (1) rules—is it right?
       (2) roles—can I feel good about this?
       (3) goals—what good will it do?
    b. keep asking: What is the fitting response?
13. Justify the option selected for recommendation.
    a. keep the patient's best interest at the center of options
    b. always provide a description of what will likely happen if this decision is made, and provide a clear action plan for each option recommended—suggestions of practical pathways.

Source: "Position of the American Dietetic Association: Ethical and Legal Issues in Nutrition, Hydration, and Feeding." *J Am Diet Assoc* 102, no. 5(2002): 716–726.

monitor legislative activity and the development of regulations, and actively promote the interests of the profession in policy formation. A legislative workshop is conducted each March in Washington, D.C., to inform members of ongoing legislation and to provide an opportunity for dietitians to meet with legislators.

In 2002, a task force of the house of delegates completed a comprehensive study of the food, nutrition, and health policies in effect.[11] Seven priority areas were recommended by the task force and became the ADA's priorities. They are: *aging, child nutrition, medical nutrition therapy, national nutrition monitoring, nutrition research, obesity, and state issues regarding recognition and scope of practice.*

Every dietitian has an obligation to be aware of policies that affect his or her practice. In addition, each individual has the opportunity of becoming a leader and influencing policy through personal awareness, active participation in communicating with policy makers, participating in national and state legislative activities, informing professional peers, and incorporating the laws and regulations into practice.

LIFELONG PROFESSIONAL DEVELOPMENT

A *Performance, Proficiency, and Value Plan* was approved and put into place by the ADA in 2002 that provided approaches toward improvement of compensation through professional development activities by ADA and by individual members.[12] Two major goals were identified that outline strategies for both groups. Goal 1 is the following: *The ADA invests in various approaches to close the gap between performance, proficiency, and value for the profession of dietetics and identifies the following strategies:*[13]

- ADA will identify educational opportunities for all levels and areas of practice to enhance value and compensation for services.
- ADA will identify tools designed to provide professional growth and development.
- ADA will identify financial opportunities for practitioners to enhance their value via grants and awards.
- ADA will identify data needed to enhance the practitioner's ability to negotiate.
- ADA will identify target audiences and alliances to market the value of the dietetic professional's services.

The second goal is the following: *Members adopt various approaches to enhance personal value.* The strategies to accomplish this goal are:[14]

- Members will commit to lifelong learning to actively engage in self-development throughout their career in dietetics.
- Members will develop personal skills and competencies for development and enhancement of practice.
- Members will use information and data to enhance understanding of performance, proficiency, and value related to the practice of dietetics.
- Members will identify skills needed to expand their scope of practice.
- Members will measure practice outcomes to demonstrate value in practice settings.

According to the House of Delegates' work group, a full discussion of actions underway to meet both goals is outlined. Many positive benefits, both professionally and through increased compensation levels, are fully anticipated.[15]

Professional development was also emphasized by Dodd and Dowling, both of whom address personal responsibility for professional performance.[16,17] Fuhrman recommends strategies to increase the credibility and visibility in clinical dietetics by being open to learning opportunities, being assertive, justifying recommendations, maintaining competency and skills in one's area of practice, and enjoying what one does![18]

Lifelong Learning

Because lifelong learning is so important to professionalism in practice, continuing professional education (CPE) has always been the cornerstone of certification of the professional dietitian. The ADA provides opportunities for lifelong learning by offering workshops, conferences, an annual meeting, self-study courses, and a professional journal. State and district association dietetic practice groups offer a variety of CPE activities as well.

An individualized plan for continued learning was implemented by the ADA in 2001 through the Professional Development Portfolio (PDP).[19] The purpose of the plan is to promote lifelong learning and provide tools to guide professionals. The plan also replaces the former requirements of reporting and gaining approval from the ADA for continuing education activities for registration maintenance. Under the PDP, the steps to follow are:

1. The individual reflects on his or her practice including strengths, needed improvements, identification of interests and trends, and then establishing short- and long-term goals.
2. The individual conducts a learning needs assessment by identifying the knowledge and skills needed to achieve the goals and define the level of CPE necessary to meet the goals.
3. The individual develops a plan to meet the goals through participation in learning activities. The plan is submitted to the ADA for approval.
4. The plan is implemented through continuing professional education.
5. The outcomes are evaluated by the individual.

Duyff points out several characteristics of the lifelong learner: ongoing curiosity, the motivation to learn, confidence in the ability to learn from others and to share, the willingness to make and learn from mistakes, persistence, flexibility in thinking, and to gather adequate information before drawing conclusions. Necessary skills include: well-developed communication methods for acquiring, processing, and transferring knowledge; determining what one needs to learn and planning toward that learning; developing information literacy and higher-order thinking skills; and honing skills for "thinking about thinking." Self-awareness, self-monitoring, positive "self-talk," and reflection are also needed, according to Duyff. In addition, she also indicated that adult learners succeed most when learning is self-directed, practical, experience based, interactive, applied, and individualized.[20]

Delivery of Learning

In planning continuing education, the type of delivery method is important in offering the material most effectively. Some professionals prefer an interactive format with small-group discussions and group presentation. Preferences are often based on relevance and timeliness, cost, accessibility, and practicality. The need for workplace programs and programs offered by different time-lines often calls for innovative programming such as that offered through distance learning.

A needs assessment survey by the CDR shows that 91 percent of RDs and DTRs have access to a personal computer; 74 percent use e-mail and 73 percent have access to the Internet.[21] A Web site was developed as an outcome of the study (www.cdr.net.org). Approved continuing professional education programs are listed on the Web site by topic. The professional development office at the ADA provides ongoing information about continuing education activities and events, and many are listed monthly in the ADA journal.

A summary of various delivery systems technologies and their characteristics is shown in Table 5–2.

Table 5–2   Characteristics of Available Delivery System Technologies

Broadcast television
- Any television set can receive the signal
- Programming times are limited; public television audience
- Programming is costly and time is needed to develop
- Communication is one way (usually no access to instructor)

Cable television
- Designed for educational access; thus, more programming time is available
- Audience is smaller; i.e., students must be subscribers
- Programming may be less costly to develop
- Existing cable companies do not serve all geographic areas

Narrowcast television (e.g., ITFS, microwave)
- Features live real-time instruction, interactive medium
- Programming times and locations are fixed
- Design can be directional or omnidirectional
- Reach can extend for a 25-mile radius
- Reception equipment and technical support are needed

Videocassette
- Students can determine viewing location and pace of learning
- Students need learning skills and independence
- Usually there is no access to the instructor at viewing time

(continues)

Table 5–2   continued

Radio/broadcast (e.g., audiocassettes, subcarrier service)
- Features easy to access, convenient, flexible format
- Specialized audiences may be served

Telephone (e.g., wired networks or dial-up services)
- Is inexpensive, easy to access, interactive, and flexible
- Audiographics can add visual support

Computer conferencing, bulletin boards, electronic campus
- Communications are asynchronous; the reach is worldwide
- Medium is compatible with available equipment/software

Interactive videodisc
- Learning stations are portable, e.g., school, worksite
- Flexible: students determine time/pace of learning
- Individualized instruction, multiple applications are possible
- Computer tools for instructional management

Satellite technology (e.g., C-Band, Ku-Band, DBS)
- Can be designed for point to multi-point transmission
- C-Band and Ku-Band use 10 to 12 foot dish/more powerful satellites allow smaller dish size
- Interference can occur from microwave or weather

Fiber optics
- Interactive medium has two-way full-motion video/audio
- Signal transmission is reliable and of superior quality
- Channels are leased on dedicated basis/equipment standards affect system capability

Digital compression/multimedia communications
- Digital video may be merged with other media
- Capable of desktop video conferencing, video production
- Technology is newer and may require new equipment, software, and applications
- Equipment standards affect system compatibility

Virtual reality
- Learning is experiential, interactive, computer-generated
- 3-D environments and simulations are featured

Key: ITFS = instructional television fixed services; DBS = direct broadcast satellite

Source: A.A. Spangler, B. Spear, and P.A. Plavcan, Dietetics Education by Distance: Current Endeavors in CAADE-Accredited/Approval Programs. Copyright The American Dietetic Association. Reprinted by permission from *Journal of The American Dietetic Association*, Vol. 95, pp. 925–929, © 1995.

Self-Responsibility for Learning

Self-direction in learning is the professional ability to engage in educational activities without external reinforcement. Individuals who are able to adapt to this behavior are those who embody some or all of the following characteristics:[22]

- Willingness to change
- Ability to identify weakness or shortcomings

- Ability to capitalize on discovered strengths and passions
- Ability to experience learning from constructive criticism by others
- Willingness to participate and be enthusiastic in all forms of learning
- Willingness to try new techniques and technologies for learning
- Willingness to invest one's time and money in learning
- Willingness to find a mentor or become one
- Volunteering and becoming active in organizations and professional groups
- Sharing learning by applying concepts immediately and discussing learning with others
- Providing feedback to instructors, mentors, and supervisors
- Assuming individual responsibility for learning
- Allowing the possibility of new career options, life paths, opportunities, and experiences

Besides maintaining and improving professional competence, there are other reasons why people participate in continuing education activities and why there may be deterrents to doing so. Several reasons and deterrents are shown in Table 5–3.

To determine the types of learning experiences that most benefit the individual, several questions may be posed for self-examination of needs (Table 5–4).

LEGAL BASIS OF PRACTICE

The practice of dietetics is directly affected by many laws and regulations that must be respected in order to avoid adverse legal consequences. Fortunately, as Derelian points out, almost all disputes that include a dietitian professional would be of

Table 5–3 Factors Influencing Continuing Professional Education

Reasons for participation in Continuing Professional Education:
- Professional development and improvement
- Professional service
- Collegial learning and interaction
- Professional commitment and reflection
- Personal benefits and job security

Deterrents in predicting participation in Continuing Professional Education:
- Disengagement and apathy for learning or career
- Costs
- Family
- Failure to see the worth and lack of benefit
- Lack of quality in offerings
- Demands of work constraints

Source: Petrillo, T. "Lifelong Learning Goals: Individual Steps that Propel the Profession of Dietetics." *J Am Diet Assoc* 103, no. 3(2003): 298–300.

Table 5–4 Questions to Determine Self Needs

What kind of learning is needed for improving performance in your current job?
Analyze your current job, talk with supervisors and discuss how to change or improve your
current job.
What is your capacity for learning and growth in a new job?
What transferable skills do you possess for a new career path?
What new skills are required for you to be qualified to contribute in a new job?
Where are your personal interests?
What career paths did you once consider?
What leisure time interests do you enjoy?
What type of a learning experience is most favorable to you and why?
What related learning opportunities lie just beyond your field of practice?
What skill sets are important to your employer?

Source: Data from Davis, J.R. "Toolbox for Reflection and Developing an Action Learning Plan: Managing Your Own." Berrett-Koehler Publisher, 2000 (10).

Petrillo, T. "Lifelong Learning Goals: Individual Steps that Propel the Profession of Dietetics." *J Am Diet Assoc* 103, no. 3(2003): 298–300.

a civil nature (contract breaches or negligence).[23] All dietitians are increasingly encouraged to carry personal liability insurance in the same way that other professions recommend of its members as a way of protecting against malpractice claims.

Regulations Affecting Dietitians

Dietitians that have licensure are under the legal system as licensure results from laws are passed in their states. State licensure laws routinely protect the title of dietitian and may also protect the scope of practice through the possibility of legal action if unqualified persons attempt to practice in dietetics.

In the present business climate, dietitians, especially those in private practice, need to be extremely astute regarding contracts for payment of services, hours of work, and conditions of work. Meerschaert points out that, in addition, one also needs to be aware of bankruptcy laws and procedures so that, if necessary, a person can act before a company that owes money is protected from their debts under the bankruptcy laws.[24] Business reorganizations and changes in administration are potential times when employees may be directly affected and therefore make it important for the individual dietitian to be aware of any or possible changes.

Price is an RD who developed expertise in legal consulting on issues primarily involving long-term care and nutrition.[25] She distributed a promotional packet to lawyers specializing in personal injury or medical malpractice suits and advertised on her Web site. By determining an hourly wage and bringing experience to bear for both written and verbal testimony when asked, dietitians may find this a challenging and rewarding career avenue.

Dietitians who work online performing activities such as sending computer analysis of food records to clients by e-mail, using e-mail to counsel patients who are traveling, conducting a chat room for groups of clients, or providing medical nutrition therapy online should be aware there are no clear guidelines for professional liability in this area. Some insurance companies are beginning to offer such liability through coverage of the scope of practice, or state licensure laws may be adequate for working with clients in state.[26] Possible liability should be investigated in any event.

Regulations Affecting Practice

The clinical dietitian may be faced with issues having to with nutritional status, hydration, and feeding of patients in unusual medical conditions or at the end of life. Many court cases have resulted from such disputes.[27] Ethical considerations are an integral part of these types of decisions as are the legal steps such as advance directives for health care by patients or their families. In any event, the role of the dietitian should be central and he or she should be guided by collaborative deliberation as part of a team and by bioethical principles. Dietitians working in long-term care facilities may also be faced with decisions about feeding for the geriatric patient. Several principles of common sense have been recommended in making such decisions: common decency, competence, commitment, communication, consultation, collaboration, consent or consensus, concern, care, compassion, and comfort.[28]

Dietitians who work in hospitals in which certification by the Joint Commission on Accreditation of Healthcare Organizations (JCAHO) is sought and maintained must be familiar with the regulations regarding patient care and safety set by this organization. Nutrition care services are regularly assessed by this organization along with all hospital services. Recently, safety goals were enacted by JCAHO concerning avoiding the use of abbreviations for treatments.[29] Dietitians are affected by these regulations because they document patient information in patients' charts and use many standard terms in providing nutrition care. Similarly, dietitians who produce educational aids or software should also avoid abbreviations that could cause confusion.

Recent federal privacy standards that protect patients' medical records and other health information provided to health plans, doctors, hospitals, and other health care providers took effect in April 2003.[30] These regulations are part of the Health Insurance Portability and Accountability Act of 1996 (HIPAA), and they apply to all health care providers. The protection of security and confidentiality of health information is the thrust of the regulations.

EVIDENCE-BASED PRACTICE

Evidence-based practice is increasingly recommended as a necessary activity leading to the best outcomes in all areas of dietetic practice. It is described as a process by which the best available data are consulted in making decisions followed by evaluation of the outcome of these decisions.[31] Dietitians need to incorporate evidence-based practice into all activities and decisions because change in practice is constant, payment for services may be dependent on outcomes, and this approach is one that ensures that decisions are sound.[32, 33] Evidence-based practice is especially vital in all clinical and patient-related activities and is critical in justifying reimbursement for medical nutrition therapy. By applying this process, dietitians will be able to successfully compete in the health care environment where proven efficiency, cost effectiveness, and sharing of outcomes are needed.[34]

SUMMARY

The professional dietitian is one who is competent in practice and continually participates in professional ongoing education. Knowledge and skills go hand in hand with personal qualities and practices including ethical practice, political awareness, understanding of the legal bases of practice, and incorporating the concept of evidence-based activities into professional practice. As the voice of authority in food and nutrition, the dietitian is a professional in every sense of the term.

DEFINITIONS

Ethics. Moral concepts of correctness and honor.
Evidence based. Action based on best data and evaluation of outcomes.
Hydration. The process of providing fluids.
Legislative action. The enactment of laws by the U.S. Congress or a state legislature.
Political awareness. Knowledge of political processes.
Profession. An occupation that involves specialized knowledge and training in which members subscribe to group beliefs and practices.
Public Policy. Course of action by a government entity for its people.
Regulations. Written directives that implement and put laws into effect.

REFERENCES

1. Gallagher, A. "Ethics in Dietetics Practice: Complicated Issues for a Complicated Time." *J Am Diet Assoc* 99, no. 11(1999): 1348.

2. "The American Dietetic Association Standards of Professional Practice for Dietetics Professionals." *J Am Diet Assoc* 98, no. 1(1998): 83–87.

3. "Code of Ethics for the Profession of Dietetics." *J Am Diet Assoc* 99, no. 1(1999): 109–113.

4. Paine, L.S. "Managing for Organizational Integrity." *Harvard Business Review* 72(1994): 106–117.

5. Waymack, M.H. "Ethical Conflicts of Interest." *J Am Diet Assoc* 103, no. 5(2003): 555–557.

6. Fornari, A. "Professional Boundary Issues in Practice." *J Am Diet Assoc* 103, no. 3(2003): 380.

7. Fornari, A. "Characteristics of Ethical Issues Versus Poor Business Practices." *J Am Diet Assoc* 103, no. 10(2002): 1380–1381.

8. "Ethical Considerations in Dietetics Practice." *J Am Diet Assoc* 100, no. 4(2000): 454.

9. "Position of the American Dietetic Association: Ethical and Legal Issues in Nutrition, Hydration, and Feeding." *J Am Diet Assoc* 102, no. 5(2002): 716–726.

10. Holler, H. "Resources for Ethical Dilemmas in Dietetics." *J Am Diet Assoc* 100, no. 5(2000): 515.

11. Discussion paper on Food, Nutrition, and Health policy. www.eatright.com/images/ leadership/nptf.pdf. American Dietetic Association, March 2002 (accessed March 15, 2004).

12. "Performance, Proficiency, and Value of the Dietetics Professional." *J Am Diet Assoc* 102, no. 9(2002): 1304–1315.

13. Ibid.

14. Ibid.

15. "Performance, Proficiency, and Value of the Dietetics Professional: An Update." *J Am Diet Assoc* 103, no. 10(2003): 1376–1379.

16. Dodd, J.L. "Look Before You Leap—But Do Leap!" *J Am Diet Assoc* 99, no. 4(1999): 422–425.

17. Dowling, R. "Role Expansion for Dietetics Professionals." *J Am Diet Assoc* 96, no. 10(1996): 1001–1002.

18. Fuhrman, M.P. "Issues Facing Dietetics Professionals: Challenges and Opportunities." *J Am Diet Assoc* 102, no. 11(2002): 1618–1620.

19. Keim, K.S., C.A. Johnson, and G.E. Gates. "Learning Needs and Continuing Professional Education Activities of Professional Development Portfolio Participants." *J Am Diet Assoc* 101, no. 6(2001): 697–702.

20. Duyff, R.L. "The Value of Lifelong Learning: Key Element in Professional Career Development." *J Am Diet Assoc* 99, no. 5(1999): 538–543.

21. Matthys, C., and M.S. Rops. "Your Input Counts: Results of the Commission on Dietetic Registration Customer Satisfaction and Needs Assessment Survey." *J Am Diet Assoc* 99, no. 7(1999): 868–870.

22. Petrillo, T. "Lifelong Learning Goals: Individual Steps That Propel the Profession of Dietetics." *J Am Diet Assoc* 103, no. 3(2003): 298–300.

23. Derelian, D. "Dietetics: Legalities, Ethics, and Eccentricities." *J Am Diet Assoc* 100, no. 5(2000): 519–523.

24. Meerschaert, C.M. "Sticky Situations: How Should You Handle Unpleasant Job Predicaments?" *Today's Dietitian* (June 2003): 27–28.

25. Price, B. "Legal Consulting: A Unique Avenue for Dietitians." *Today's Dietitian* (June 2001): 24–26.

26. Grieger, L. "Working Online: Are You Covered?" *Today's Dietitian* (November 2001): 41–42.

27. Holler, H. "Resources for Ethical Dilemmas in Dietetics." *J Am Diet Assoc* 100, no. 5(2000): 515.

28. McDermott, A.Y., A. Shevitz, S. Must, R. Roubenoff, and S. Gorback. "Ethical and Legal Issues in Nutrition Support of the Geriatric Patient." *Nutr Clin Prac* (2003): 18:21–36.

29. Phillips, M.W. "Avoiding Medical Errors: JCAHO Documentation Requirements." *J Am Diet Assoc* 104, no. 2(2004): 171–173.

30. "Protecting the Privacy of Patient's Health Information. www.hhs.gov/ocu/hipaa, [Health and Human Services] (accessed March 20, 2004).

31. Shanklin, C. "Evidence-Based Practice: Practice Based on Evidence, Right?" *ADA Times* 1, no. 3(2003): 1, 3.

32. Vaughan, L.A., and C.K. Manning. "Meeting the Challenges of Dietetics Practice with Evidence-Based Decisions." *J Am Diet Assoc* 104, no. 2(2004): 282–284.

33. Franz, M.J. "The Lenna Frances Cooper Memorial Lecture—The Future of Clinical Dietetics: Evidence, Outcomes, and Reimbursement." *J Am Diet Assoc* 103, no. 8 (2003): 977–981.

34. Smith, R. "Expanding Medical Nutrition Therapy: An Argument for Evidence-Based Practices." *Journal of the American Dietetics Association* 103, no. 3 (2003): 313–314.

PART III

Areas of Practice

CHAPTER 6

The Dietitian in Clinical Practice

"The dietetic practitioner interacts with complex beings who eat food rather than nutrients. The psychosocial aspects of diet modification may therefore determine ultimate clinical usefulness and ethical practice."[1]

Outline

- Introduction
- Employment Settings of Clinical Dietitians
  — Managed health care
- Organization of Clinical Nutritional Services
- Responsibilities in Clinical Dietetics
  — Nutrition care process
  — Medical nutrition therapy
- Major Functions and Time Involvement
- The Clinical Nutrition Service Team
  — Clinical nutrition managers/chief clinical dietitians
  — Clinical dietitians
  — Dietetic technicians
  — Dietetic assistants
- Clinical Dietetics Outlook
- Summary

INTRODUCTION

The discipline of clinical dietetics originated in 1899 when *dietitian* was defined by the American Home Economic Association as "individuals with a knowledge of food who provide diet therapy for the medical profession." Until 1917, dietitians were affiliated with this association, but after 1917 they belonged to the newly formed American Dietetic Association (ADA).[2]

The earliest dietitians worked primarily in hospitals or were associated with food assistance programs. During the 1930s and 1940s, dietitians became involved either in food production and food service or in the planning and provision of diets for special medical needs. The title *therapeutic dietitian* was used to describe the person who provided food for medical reasons, such as to prevent a nutrient deficiency or to help with the treatment of disease.[3] Examples of early diet therapy include the Sippy diet that used milk and cream to treat ulcers and the Kempner rice diet used to treat hypertension; each was named for the physician who designed it.

As the dietitian's role in the hospital became one of providing specialized care and modifying diets to treat various medical conditions, the title *clinical dietitian* replaced the former *therapeutic dietitian*.

In the early 1970s, reports of widespread malnutrition among hospitalized patients helped to increase the visibility of the clinical dietitian.[4] Rather than providing diet therapy as ordered by physicians, clinical dietitians began to take a more active role in screening and monitoring the provision of nutrition support. Development of individual nutrition care plans became important functions of clinical dietitians. As the role of diet in the etiology of chronic diseases became better defined, clinical dietitians began to spend a greater percentage of their time participating in the prevention of diseases such as heart disease, cancer, and diabetes.

EMPLOYMENT SETTINGS OF CLINICAL DIETITIANS

In 2002, 79 percent of both RDs and DTRs reported they were currently employed in dietetics.[5] In fact, this high percentage of dietitians and dietetic technicians who were working in the field of dietetics reflects the diversity of job opportunities. Tables 6–1 and 6–2 show the primary employment settings.[6] Fifty-four percent of RDs and 62 percent of DTRs were employed in the clinical areas of practice of acute care/inpatient, ambulatory care, and long-term care. The findings and earlier membership surveys with similar findings indicate stability in employment areas.

The three primary areas of clinical practice are:

1. Acute care/inpatient
   • hospitals

Table 6–1   Practice Area, Primary Position

	RDs (%)	DTRs (%)
Clinical nutrition—acute care/inpatient	28	41
Clinical nutrition—ambulatory care	14	1
Clinical nutrition—long-term care	12	20
Community	11	10
Food and nutrition management	13	20
Consultation and business	11	2
Education and research	6	1

Base: 9,220 practicing RDs; 1,498 practicing DTRs.

Source: Rogers, D. "Report on the ADA 2002 Dietetics Compensation and Benefits Survey." *J Am Diet Assoc* 163, no. 2(2003): 243–255.

2. Ambulatory care
   - hospital outpatient departments
   - clinics
   - outpatient care centers
3. Long-term care
   - nursing homes
   - assisted living facilities
   - Alzheimer's units

Table 6–2   Highest Incidence Positions—RDs

	RDs (%)
Clinical dietitian	16
Clinical dietitian, specialist—renal	3
Outpatient dietitian, general	4
Outpatient dietitian, specialist—diabetes	4
Outpatient dietitian, specialist—renal	3
Clinical dietitian, long-term care	12
Women, Infants, and Children nutritionist	5
Public health nutritionist	3
Director of food and nutrition services	5
Clinical nutrition manager	4
Private practice dietitian—patient/client nutrition care	3

Base: 9,220 practicing RDs.

Source: Rogers, D. "Report on the ADA 2002 Dietetics Compensation and Benefits Survey." *J Am Diet Assoc* 163, no. 2(2003): 243–255.

Managed Health Care

Many hospitals and health care institutions are operated under managed care organizations that have become a major means of the delivery of health care in the United States. The cost and access to health care are major reasons for this trend. Health maintenance organizations (HMO) are the primary type of managed care plans dietitians are likely to be associated with, although there are others such as integrated delivery systems or groups of delivery systems.[7] The basic concepts of managed care are that medical care will be provided in exchange for a set fee, a primary physician is designated, and that prevention of disease is stressed as a means of controlling costs before conditions require expensive treatment.[8]

ORGANIZATION OF CLINICAL NUTRITION SERVICES

Clinical nutrition services may be organized in a variety of ways, depending on the setting. Clinical nutrition services in most hospitals are managed by a clinical nutrition manager, the director of clinical nutrition, or the chief clinical dietitian (see Figure 6–1a). Typically, the chief clinical dietitian reports to an individual whose primary responsibilities are food service and the financial management of the entire food and nutrition department. In some instances, clinical dietetics may be organized as a separate department that reports to an executive or administrator with other patient care responsibilities such as nursing or pharmacy (see Figure 6–1b). There are advantages and disadvantages to both types of organization. Combining clinical nutrition with food services can facilitate communication regarding patient food choices and menus. By contrast, having clinical nutrition as a separate department may increase visibility as an important patient care service unit distinct from food service.

RESPONSIBILITIES IN CLINICAL DIETETICS

Nutrition Care Process

The Quality Management Committee of the ADA developed a nutrition care process (NCP) and model that was adopted by the house of delegates in 2003.[9] The purpose of the planning model was "for implementation and dissemination to the dietetics profession and the association for the enhancement of the practice of dietetics."[10] The NCP is defined as systematic problem-solving methods that dietetic professionals use to critically think and make decisions to address nutrition-

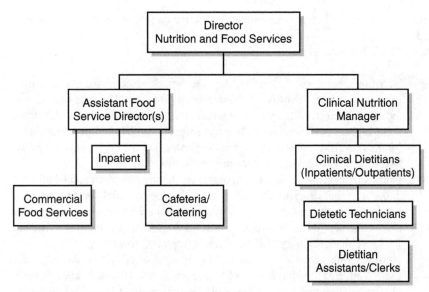

a. Clinical Nutrition within a Nutrition Department

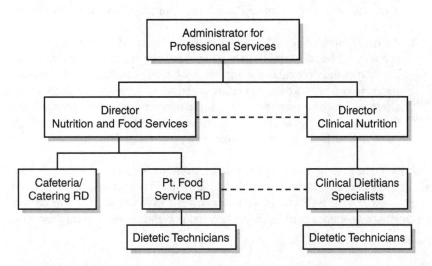

b. Clinical Nutrition within a Separate Department

Figure 6–1A and B Examples of Nutrition and Food Service Organizational Charts. *Sources:* Example A is courtesy of The Methodist Hospital, Houston, Texas. Example B is courtesy of Nutrition Center, Arkansas Children's Hospital, Little Rock, Arkansas.

related problems and to provide safe and effective quality nutrition care (see Figure 6–2).

The NCP has four steps:

1. Nutrition assessment. In the first step, the dietetic professional obtains information in order to identify nutrition-related problems. The type of data collected includes the dietary history with detailed nutrient intake, health status using anthropometric and biochemical measures, and functional and behavioral status. If the initial assessment indicates that the problem is not nutrition related, the remaining steps are not followed.
2. Nutrition diagnosis. This step encompasses the identification and labeling of conditions that describe the occurrence, risk, or potential for developing a nutritional problem that dietetics professionals are responsible for treating independently. When possible, a nutrition diagnostic statement is written in PES (problem, etiology, and signs and symptoms) format.
3. Nutrition intervention. An intervention is a set of activities and materials used to address the identified problem or problems. Two steps are involved: (1) formulating and determining a plan of action, and (2) implementing the plan. When implemented, the dietitian communicates the plan, carries out the plan, and collects data toward continuation or modification of the plan of care.
4. Nutrition monitoring and evaluation. In the monitoring step, the patient/client/group status is reviewed and measured at a specific follow-up point. Evaluation then provides a comparison of current findings with previous status, intervention goals, or a reference standard. In this process, the client progress is monitored to determine if the intervention is or is not changing the client's behavior or status. The outcome indicators are selected and applied and the findings are compared with previous goals or standards.

It should be noted that NCP is the broader, over-arching guide to a full spectrum of nutrition care, and medical nutrition therapy (MNT) is a process for delivery of nutrition care.[11] The NCP provides the steps a dietitian would use in delivering this therapy but also guides nutrition education and preventive nutrition care services.

Medical Nutrition Therapy

The term *medical nutrition therapy* arose with the national attention on health care reform and growth of managed care, with its emphasis on cost-effectiveness and financial management of services. It is increasingly important to show that nutrition services are beneficial and essential in providing care and that nutrition services should be reimbursed by insurers and other third-party payers.

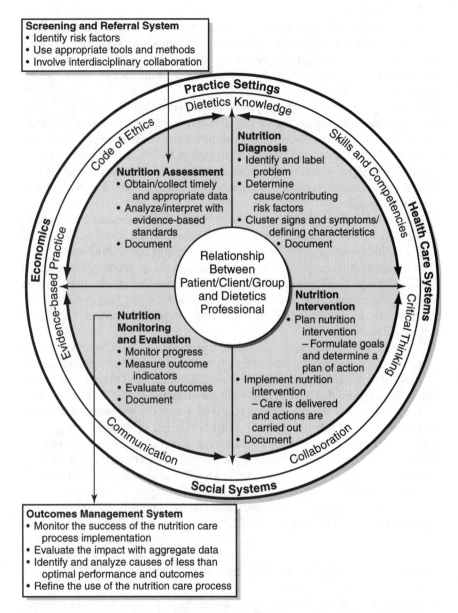

Screening and Referral System
- Identify risk factors
- Use appropriate tools and methods
- Involve interdisciplinary collaboration

Practice Settings

Dietetics Knowledge

Code of Ethics

Skills and Competencies

Nutrition Diagnosis
- Identify and label problem
- Determine cause/contributing risk factors
- Cluster signs and symptoms/ defining characteristics
- Document

Nutrition Assessment
- Obtain/collect timely and appropriate data
- Analyze/interpret with evidence-based standards
- Document

Economics

Evidence-based Practice

Health Care Systems

Critical Thinking

Relationship Between Patient/Client/Group and Dietetics Professional

Nutrition Intervention
- Plan nutrition intervention
  – Formulate goals and determine a plan of action
- Implement nutrition intervention
  – Care is delivered and actions are carried out
- Document

Nutrition Monitoring and Evaluation
- Monitor progress
- Measure outcome indicators
- Evaluate outcomes
- Document

Communication

Collaboration

Social Systems

Outcomes Management System
- Monitor the success of the nutrition care process implementation
- Evaluate the impact with aggregate data
- Identify and analyze causes of less than optimal performance and outcomes
- Refine the use of the nutrition care process

Figure 6–2 ADA Nutrition Care Process and Model. *Source:* Lacey, K., and E. Pritchett. Nutrition Care Process and Model. *J Am Diet Assoc* 2003; 103(8): 1061–1071.

MNT is vital to the medical management of acute and chronic diseases, lowering costs by speeding recovery and reducing complications. Fewer hospitalizations, shorter hospital stays, and diminished need for other treatments are the results. In preventing disease development, MNT reduces risk of disease, maintains health, and improves quality of life.[12]

Recognition of MNT was established in 2002 when Congress passed a bill establishing Medicare coverage for nutritional management in the treatment of, specifically, diabetes and renal disease.[13] A focus of legislative efforts by the ADA is to extend MNT to cardiovascular and other disease conditions; however, dietitians use the MNT process for many nutrition-related conditions and diseases despite the lack of coverage for nutrition services by insurers. A model of MNT in practice is shown in Figure 6–3.

MNT involves the assessment of the nutritional status of patients with a condition, illness, or injury that puts them at risk. The assessment involves review and analysis of the medical and diet history, laboratory values, and anthropometric measures. Based on the assessment, nutrition modalities most appropriate to manage the condition or treat the illness or injury are chosen. These include diet modification and counseling leading to the development of a personal diet plan to achieve nutritional goals and desired health outcomes and specialized nutrition therapies in specified conditions.

The value of MNT has been reported in several studies: hypercholesterolemia,[14] weight loss,[15] hypertension,[16] and hyperlipidemia.[17] In a 2003 position paper, the ADA stated the following: "It is the position of the American Dietetic Association that the application of MNT and lifestyle counseling as a part of the nutrition care process is an integral component of the medical treatment for management of specific disease states and conditions and should be the initial step in the management of these situations. If optimal control cannot be achieved with MNT, then the association promotes a team approach to care for clients receiving concurrent MNT and pharmacotherapy and encourages active collaboration among dietetics professionals and other members of the health care team."[18]

The ADA has a number of resources available for practitioners using MNT and the Medicare system for access to MNT.[19]

MAJOR FUNCTIONS AND TIME INVOLVEMENT

A profile of the amount of time spent by clinical dietitians at the functions they perform was reported by Shanklin and colleagues (1988).[20] In this study, dietitians spent 51 percent of their time performing client-related activities, 10 percent in managerial functions, 1 percent in professional activities, 5 percent in nonprofessional activities, and 20 percent in transit time.

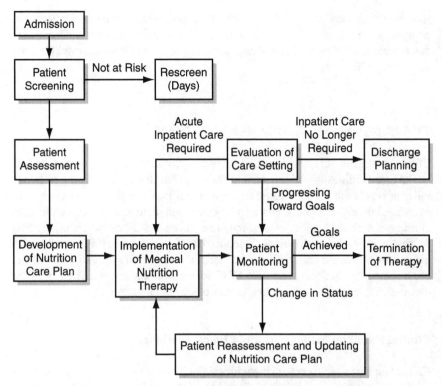

Figure 6–3 Provision of Medical Nutrition Therapy for Hospitalized Patients. *Source:* Reprinted from the American Society for Parental and Enteral Nutrition (A.S.P.E.N.). "Guidelines for the Use of Parenteral and Enteral Nutrition in Adult and Pediatric Patients." *Journal of Parenteral and Enteral Nutrition* 17 (suppl 4) 1993:1SA–525A.

In regard to client-related activities, the major functions performed were documentation of nutritional care (16 percent), preliminary nutritional screening (11 percent), health team conferences (10 percent), and nutritional care evaluation and reassessment (10 percent). Patient diagnosis and the complexity of the dietary modifications influence the time required by dietitians to perform these functions. In general, dietitians spend more time providing clinical services to patients with diagnoses involving the endocrine (e.g., diabetes) or renal (kidney) systems.

The type of diet order also influences the amount of time a dietitian spends in patient care. Calorie-controlled diabetic diets, modified mineral content for cardiac conditions, and individualized diets for specific patient needs are extremely time consuming. The calculation and design of complex dietary modifications is especially time-consuming for dietitians caring for pediatric patients. Pediatric patients may require more frequent monitoring. The patient's growth and energy requirements must also be factored into the diet plan, and for some, modifications may need to be made daily.

THE CLINICAL NUTRITION SERVICE TEAM

Clinical nutrition services may be provided by a number of team members in health care facilities. Inpatient nutritional care in hospitals is usually the responsibility of persons in several positions: clinical nutrition managers/chief clinical dietitians, clinical dietitians, dietetic technicians, and dietetic assistants. Outpatient clinics and ambulatory care centers may use all four positions but are more likely to employ only clinical dietitians. Extended care facilities and HMOs or physician offices may have clinical dietitians on staff; however, more often these facilities use a consulting dietitian to provide MNT for patients and clients. The consulting dietitian may be in private practice or part of a group practice.

Clinical Nutrition Managers/Chief Clinical Dietitians

Clinical nutrition managers or chief clinical dietitians are primarily responsible for directing the activities of clinical dietitians, dietetic technicians, and dietetic assistants. Major tasks performed include hiring of clinical nutrition employees, evaluating employee job performance, providing in-service and on-the-job training, reviewing productivity reports, writing job descriptions, scheduling employees, developing policies and procedures, designing performance standards, and developing and implementing goals and objectives of the department.[21] The clinical nutrition manager is also responsible for communicating with the staffs of other departments and administration. Ultimately, the clinical nutrition manager ensures that performance is actually accomplished to achieve the goals and objectives of the department.

Clinical Dietitians

The primary responsibility of the clinical dietitian is to provide nutritional care for patients. Clinical dietitians in hospitals are involved in nutritional screening of patients to determine the presence of or risk of developing malnutrition, performing nutritional assessments, and developing nutrition care plans. Clinical nutrition services may be provided to general patient care units or may be based on a medical specialization (e.g., critical care or diabetes education). Clinical dietitians are important members of the health care team because they consult and collaborate with physicians, pharmacists, nurses, social workers, chaplains, and others when providing nutritional care.

Clinical dietitians are the source of authoritative knowledge about MNT and patient education. They routinely communicate with other disciplines regarding developments in MNT and patient education through in-service teams, rounds, and multidisciplinary patient care conferences.

Successful clinical dietitians in acute health care facilities must also be able to apply managerial concepts to provide effective nutritional care. Management tasks often performed by clinical dietitians include in-service training, on-the-job training, employee interviews and evaluations, writing job descriptions, planning cycle menus, and evaluating the quality of patient food.[22]

Clinical dietitians working in settings other than acute health care facilities tend to be involved in a wider range of tasks. Their responsibilities often include more managerial and administrative tasks similar to the duties of a clinical manager. In addition, they may provide more preventive nutrition therapy through modification of lifestyle.

Typical responsibilities of three different levels of clinical dietitians in a large, acute care hospital are shown in Table 6–3, with an indication of the knowledge, skill, and experience required of each in Table 6–4.

Clinical dietitians may be members of one or more dietetic practice groups. Besides dietitians in general clinical practice, these may include gerontological nutritionist, dietetics in developmental and psychiatric disorders, oncology nutrition, renal dietitians, pediatric nutrition, diabetes care and support, dietitians in nutrition support, perinatal nutrition, HIV/AIDS, and others. The diversity of specialty and subspecialty areas of practice reflects the broad range of interests and opportunities open to the clinical dietitian.

Dietetic Technicians

The primary responsibility of the dietetic technician in the clinical setting is to assist the clinical dietitian. Typically, the major functions performed are gathering data for nutritional screening and assigning a level of risk for malnutrition according to predetermined criteria. They may help with nutritional assessments by gathering laboratory and anthropometric data, collecting and analyzing nutrient intake information, obtaining nutritional histories, and reviewing medical histories. Dietetic technicians may administer nourishment and dietary supplements for patients and monitor patient tolerance. They may also provide information to help patients select

Table 6–3   Clinical Dietitian Responsibilities

Function	Staff	Senior	Specialist
Nutritional screening	X	X	X
Nutritional assessments/care plans:			
Diet instructions	X	X	X
General patients	X	X	X
Critical care/complex patients		X	X
Diet calculations, eating plans, menu checking, evaluation of meal service	X	X	X
Evaluates nutrient intake and provides follow-up care	X	X	X
Directs activities of dietetic technicians and dietetic assistants	X	X	X
Provides clinical inservices to dietitians, dietetic technicians, and dietitian assistants	X	X	X
Participates in performance evaluation of dietetic technician and dietetic assistants	X	X	X
Medical team rounds and multidisciplinary team meetings	X	X	X
Evaluation of clinical monitors for quality management	X	X	X
On-call duties (weekend/week night)	X	X	X
Clinical nutrition committee membership	X	X	X
Clinical responsibility in focus area—patient education or assessment		X	X
Maintains reference in area of clinical focus		X	X
Revises standards of care and clinical procedures		X	X
Conducts peer review of clinical dietitian chart notes		X	X
Trains new staff interns		X	X
Clinical responsibility in area of specialization			X
Provides updates in specialization area			X
Participates in research and presents findings			X
Scheduling dietitian coverage in absence of supervisor			X
Chairs clinical committees		cochairs	cochairs

Source: Courtesy of The Methodist Hospital, Houston, Texas, 1998.

Table 6–4   Knowledge, Skill, and Experience Requirements for Clinical Dietitians

Function	Staff	Senior	Specialist
Registered dietitian (the ADA)	Yes	Yes	Yes
Licensure	Yes	Yes	Yes
Clinical experience (years)	Entry	3	5
Advanced knowledge and certification	No	No	Yes
Outside continuing education hours	No	Yes	Yes

Source: Courtesy of The Methodist Hospital, Houston, Texas, 1998.

menus and give simple diet instructions. Dietetic technicians maintain a high level of knowledge of nutritional care. Management responsibilities of dietetic technicians may include supervision of dietetic assistants.

Dietetic Assistants

Dietetic assistants help the clinical dietitian and/or dietetic technician in some of the more routine aspects of nutritional care. They are often responsible for processing diet orders, checking menus against standards, setting up standard nourishments, and tallying special food requests. Dietetic assistants may also help distribute and pick up inpatient menus and pass and collect trays. They may be involved in evaluating patient food satisfaction and gathering food records to be used to evaluate nutrient intake.

CLINICAL DIETETICS OUTLOOK

Changes in health care occur rapidly. Within the next several years, health care services now provided only at community hospitals are expected to be provided at alternative sites. It has been projected that future health care systems will be dispersed over wide geographic areas. More health care may even be offered through telecommunications from central sites. Ambulatory care centers are expected to replace, in large part, the typical hospital.[23] These changes are affecting, and will continue to affect, the practice of clinical dietitians.

In the future, employment of dietitians by hospitals is expected to grow slowly because a greater number of hospital food service operations will be contracted to private companies who will provide their own dietitians. By contrast, employment opportunities in rehabilitation centers, nursing homes, and residential care centers will grow as the population continues to age.[24]

By 2005, the settings with the greatest projected employment demand for clinical dietitians will include physician offices (54 percent), offices of other health care professionals (63 percent), nursing and home health care facilities (9 percent), and residential care (129 percent).[25]

The future roles of clinical dietitians can be expanded by developing new skills and competencies.[26] Advanced training and education, cross-training in allied health areas for multicompetency, department management, counseling skills, multicultural training, and computer technical competency are all considered valuable assets for expanded roles. Employment opportunities are expected to increase as clinical dietitians expand their role into areas providing more community-based care and preventive care. Efforts that increase access to health care will also increase employment opportunities for clinical dietitians. By emphasizing primary care and prevention through promotion of healthy lifestyles, clinical dietitians can expand their role and remain an important health care provider in the future.

SUMMARY

The clinical dietitian plays a major role in helping persons during illness through nutrition interventions and MNT. Equally important is helping individuals prevent the onset of chronic disease by the application of optimal nutrition practices throughout life. A current challenge for the professional practitioner in clinical dietetics is the expansion of MNT with cost-effectiveness data and demonstration of quality practice, and increased recognition of the importance of nutritional care by insurers and third-party payers.

Even though employment may move outside the hospital or clinic, the services provided by the clinical dietitian will remain vital to the health and well-being of people in illness and injury.

DEFINITIONS

Ambulatory Care Center. A health care facility in which nonhospitalized patients are treated.

Clinical Dietetics. The area of practice in which persons with illness or injury are treated by using nutrition assessment, planning, and implementation of nutrition care plans.

Clinical Nutrition Services. Activities provided in the practice of clinical dietetics, such as medical nutrition therapy and counseling.

Diet Therapy. Treatment by diet; this term is now replaced by clinical nutrition therapy or medical nutrition therapy.

Extended Care Facility. Institution that "extends" health care beyond the acute-care setting; when long-term care is needed.

Managed Care Organization. Group providing comprehensive health care services in which access, cost, and quality are controlled by direct intervention before or during service.

Medical Nutrition Therapy. The application of nutrition in the management of illness or injury.

Outpatient Clinic. Treatment area of a hospital or health care facility in which patients are treated on an outpatient basis.

REFERENCES

1. Coulston, A.M., and C.L. Rock. "A Summary of the Current State of Knowledge in Clinical Nutrition and Dietetic Practice: Suggestions for Future Research in Dietetic Practice and Implications for Health Care." In *The Research Agenda for Dietitians.* ADA Conference Proceedings. Chicago: The American Dietetic Association (1993): 1–24.

2. Cooper, L.F. "The Dietitian and Her Profession." *J Am Diet Assoc* 14(1938): 751–758.

3. Huyck, I., and M.M. Rowe. *Managing Clinical Nutrition Services.* Rockville, MD: Aspen Publishers, 1990.

4. Butterworth, E. "The Skeleton in the Hospital Closet." *Nutrition Today* 9 (1974): 4.

5. Rogers, D. "Report on the ADA 2002 Dietetics Compensation and Benefits Survey." *J Am Diet Assoc* 103, no. 2(2003): 243–255.

6. Ibid.

7. Laramee, S.H. "Nutrition Services in Managed Care: New Paradigms for Dietitians." *J Am Diet Assoc* 96(1996): 335–336.

8. Fielder, K.M. "Managed Health Care: Understanding the Role of the Nutrition Professional." *J Am Diet Assoc* 93(1993): 1111–1112.

9. Lacey, K., and E. Pritchett. "Nutrition Care Process and Model: ADA Adopts Road Map to Quality Care and Outcomes Management." *J Am Diet Assoc* 103, no. 8(2003): 1061–1071.

10. Ibid.

11. Ibid.

12. ADA. "Position of the American Dietetic Association: Nutrition Services in Managed Care. *J Am Diet Assoc* 102, no. 10(2003): 1471–1478.

13. Ibid.

14. Delehanty, L.M., L.M. Sonnenberg, D. Hayden, and D.M. Nathan. "Clinical and Cost Outcomes of Medical Nutrition Therapy for Hypercholesterolemia: A Controlled Study." *J Am Diet Assoc* 101, no. 9(2001): 1012–1016.

15. Splett, P.L., L.L. Roth-Yousey, and J.L. Vogelzang. "Medical Nutrition Therapy for the Prevention and Treatment of Unintentional Weight Loss in Residential Healthcare Facilities." *J Am Diet Assoc* 103, no. 3(2003): 352–362.

16. ADA Position Paper. "Position of the American Dietetic Association: Integration of Medical Nutrition and Pharmacotherapy." *J Am Diet Assoc* 103, no. 10(2003): 1363–1370.

17. Ibid.

18. Ibid.

19. "Celebrating the Significance of the Medicare MNT Benefit—One Year Anniversary." *Diet Pract* (Winter 2002): 1–2.

20. Shanklin, C.W., H.N. Hernandez, R.M. Gould, and M.A. Gorman. "Results of a Statewide Time Study in Texas." *J Am Diet Assoc* 88(1988): 38–43.

21. Digh, E.W., and R.P. Dowdy. "A Survey of Management Tasks Completed by Clinical Dietitians in the Practice Setting." *J Am Diet Assoc* 94(1994): 1381–1384.

22. Ibid.

23. Brylinsky, C. "Shifting Clinical Dietetics to New Markets." *Clinic Nutr Manager Newsletter* 15(1995): 4–5.

24. Kornblum, T.H. "Professional Demand for Dietitians and Nutritionists in the Year 2005." *J Am Diet Assoc* 94(1994): 21–22.

25. Ibid.

26. Parks, S.C., P.A. Fitz, J.O. Maillet, P. Babjak, and B. Mitchell. "Challenging the Future of Dietetics Education and Credentialing—Dialogue, Discovery, and Directions: A Summary of the 1994 Future Search Conference." *J Am Diet Assoc* 95(1995): 598–606.

CHAPTER 7

Management in Food and Nutrition Systems

"Knowledge of food and management skills is essential to most areas of practice in dietetics. Many dietetic practice groups, including those in clinical nutrition, community nutrition and business practice, routinely translate nutrition science into food choices *for specific audiences.*"[1]

Outline

- Introduction
- Areas of Employment
  - Food service in acute care
  - Food service in long-term care
  - Food service in noninstitutional settings
  - School nutrition programs
  - Clinical nutrition management
  - Commercial food services
  - Further areas of opportunity
- Roles and Responsibilities
- Standards of Professional Practice
- Characteristics of Successful Food and Nutrition Managers
- Career Ladder Opportunities
- Summary

INTRODUCTION

Food and food service are prominent in the history of the profession of dietetics. One of the main purposes of the first organizing meeting of the American Dietetic Association (ADA) was to discuss ways of meeting food shortages during World War I. Many of the first members of the association served overseas, feeding hospitalized soldiers and people living under wartime conditions. Cooking schools, scientists who produced the first tables of food values, early day soup kitchens, and school lunch programs were among the forerunners of institutions that fed the public.[2]

Food service in hospitals was the primary focus of the first dietitians. During the 1890s, food service in hospitals was managed by the chef, the housekeeper, or the nursing department. In the early 1900s, however, many dietitians were in charge of dietary departments and had the responsibility for all food service plus teaching nurses and providing diet therapy for patients with metabolic diseases. Hospital dietitians dealt with budgets, department organization, personnel management, and quality food service. Nutrition was recognized as an aspect of medicine, and food prescriptions were handled as apothecary compounds, thus creating a demand for special diet kitchens. The hospital dietitian had the same status as the superintendent of nurses and was recognized as the nutrition expert.[3]

Dietitians with food service management responsibilities became members of the Food Administration section in the ADA, and their practice was referred to as "administrative dietetics." The terminology now used is food service systems management or management in food and nutrition systems.

Spears defines the manager as "one who is responsible for people and organizational resources and possesses management skills including technical, human, and conceptual."[4] In this chapter, the focus is on the dietitian in food service management and the manager in clinical services.

AREAS OF EMPLOYMENT

The majority of dietitians begin their career in clinical practice. About half of those beyond entry level (10 years or more of practice), however, are employed in food and nutrition management.

Dietitians in food service management typically affiliate with four ADA dietetic practice groups: Management in Food and Nutrition Systems, Dietitians in Business and Communication, School Nutrition Services, and Food and Culinary Professionals. In addition, clinical managers may belong to the Clinical Nutrition Management group. Management dietitians may be identified through a wide range of titles. Taylor identified titles of coordinator, specialist, and executive dietitian.[5] Among more traditional titles, Liu found position titles of directors/associate directors of food and nutrition services, directors of clinical nutrition, directors of multiunit services, and food/nutrition consultants.[6] Molt described titles such as director, chief, or chief administrator among dietitians working in hospital food service, school food service, and college and university residence halls.[7]

The 1990 role delineation studies for registered dietitians and dietetic technicians categorized practice areas by work settings.[8] The categories included food service in acute care, food service in long-term care, and food service in the noninstitutional population. To encompass the broader management area, clinical nutrition management, commercial food services, and school nutrition have been added to this list. A brief discussion of each of these areas follows.

Food Service in Acute Care

Food service in acute care is described as food service in hospitals or similar health care institutions in which patients receive short-term medical treatment, usually 1 to 5 days. Several characteristics of this type of food service are:

1. fast turnover of patients with day-to-day fluctuations in the number of meals prepared and served
2. special diets requiring different types of food preparation (in some instances, as many as 30 to 50 percent of all patients will require special or modified diets)
3. selective menus for patients, increasing the number of food items prepared
4. multiple serving systems in an institution, such as individual tray service for patients, cafeteria service and vending for hospital personnel and the public, and catering for hospital staff
5. various types of food service for patients.

In some institutions, food is prepared in bulk, then pre-portioned and held until the time of meal service when it is reheated and served. In others, food is prepared centrally just before meal service and either portioned individually or sent in bulk to patient areas of individual service. In each system, the dietitian has overall responsibility for food production and service or may share this responsibility with chefs and managers. Whatever the scope of his or her responsibility, the dietitian must be knowledgeable in food production techniques, food purchasing, safety and sanitation, strategic planning, human relations, communications, and managerial skills.

Food Service in Long-Term Care

The provision of food for clients in nursing homes, extended care facilities, and correctional institutions is included in this category.[9] Food service in these types of institutions differs from that in acute care in that clients are long term and are usually served in group settings. Central food production and few special diets are the norm because most of the long-term clients will be following a normal, healthy eating pattern. The food service, especially in smaller nursing homes and extended care facilities, may be managed by a dietetic technician or by a certified dietary manager under the direction of a dietitian-consultant. In correctional institutions, the day-to-day management is often provided by nonprofessionals under the direction of a dietitian-consultant when one is available. All aspects of food service management are equally important in long-term care as in the hospital, with the added necessity of ensuring nutritional adequacy and acceptability over longer periods of time. Federal and state regulations relate to the provision of food services to clients in almost all long-term facilities, and must be followed for the institution to receive funding and provide quality care. The qualifications for the food service manager are also stated in the regulations.

Food Service in Noninstitutional Settings

This type of food service includes colleges and universities, employee cafeterias, and business and commercial enterprises. These types of food service organizations vary in several ways, and may be profit or nonprofit. Generally, those serving the public will be for-profit while those in schools or in businesses providing employee food services will be nonprofit. Clients choose to patronize the food services offered, and the types of food services may vary widely. A college or university, for instance, may offer cafeteria, dining room, restaurant, catering, and/or vending services. School and employee food service is often by cafeteria service along with vending and dining room service. The dietitian's responsibility is to provide food that is safe and acceptable to the customers, meets financial expectations, and promotes good nutrition.

School Nutrition Programs

School nutrition programs, offering either lunch, breakfast, or both, are available to more than 90 percent of all students. About 25 million students from preschool to grade 12 are fed daily.[10] The programs are administered and partially funded by the federal government, and they must meet specific guidelines for nutritional quality of meals and student eligibility. Free meals are provided based on the family economic status. The emphasis is on long-term health benefits for children through establishing good eating habits. A position statement supporting school nutrition programs is the following:

> It is the position of the American Dietetic Association, the Society for Nutrition Education, and the American School Food Service Association that

comprehensive nutrition services must be provided to all of the nation's preschool through grade twelve students. These nutrition services shall be integrated with a coordinated, comprehensive school health program and implemented through a school nutrition policy. The policy should link comprehensive sequential nutrition education; access to and promotion of child nutrition programs providing nutritious meals and snacks in the school environment; and family, community, and health services' partnerships supporting positive health outcomes for all children.[11]

Dietitians in school nutrition programs need both managerial and nutrition education skills. Many in this career area affiliate with the School Nutrition Services dietetic practice group and also the American School Food Service Association.

The National Food Service Management Institute conducted research to determine the functions and tasks of school nutrition managers. The job functions rated most important were program accountability, sanitation and safety, customer service, equipment use and care, and food production. The manager in a school food service program has responsibilities in at least seven other areas: nutrition and menu planning, food procurement, food acceptability, financial management, marketing, personnel management, and professional development.[12]

Clinical Nutrition Management

Clinical nutrition management refers to the activities of practitioners in hospitals and health care institutions who develop and operate systems that successfully meet the nutritional needs of patients.[13] This may include the responsibility for one or more units and the supervision of other professionals in clinical areas. The clinical manager performs many of the same management functions as the food service dietitian: management of human, financial, and material resources. The clinical dietitian who progresses from an entry-level position to a management position will normally have 5 to 10 years or more of experience and will not be involved in day-to-day activities directly related to patient care.

Commercial Food Services

Shanklin and Dowling describe commercial food service as retail and hospitality food service establishments that prepare food for immediate consumption on-or-off the premises.[14] The types of establishments employing dietitians include independent restaurants, casual/family dining restaurants, and fine dining restaurants. Supermarket chains, limited service (fast-food) chains, and hotel chains also have high potential for dietetic services. Five specific areas of need in these institutions are nutrition education, healthful menu planning, recipe and menu analysis, marketing, and quality control.

Lechowich and Soto reported a study of opportunities in commercial food services from the industry standpoint and found that although the opportunities exist, relatively few dietitians are employed in these areas. Skills in areas such as public relations, communications, marketing, and purchasing are usually expected; therefore, additional training and experience are often needed by the dietitian to be fully qualified for these roles.[15]

Further Areas of Opportunity

Further opportunities for dietitians in food service management include positions in food corporations (research, consumer affairs, communications), disaster planning centers, military bases, homeless shelters and food distribution centers, worldwide religious ministries and government food programs, and academic units with food/nutrition/hospitality programs. Many dietitians are employed in contract food service companies that provide management services for profit. Hospitals, colleges and universities, schools, employee cafeterias in businesses, hotels and restaurants, and health care institutions may contract with a company that manages the food services for a negotiated fee. The companies hire and often train their own personnel including dietitian-managers.

ROLES AND RESPONSIBILITIES

Three major studies, conducted by the ADA, describe the roles and responsibilities of dietitians in areas of practice. The first was the Role Delineation Study (1990), followed by the Commission on Dietetic Registration Practice Audit (1996) and the Educational Competencies Steering Committee on Competencies (1997).

In the Role Delineation Study, the average amount of time spent in activities related to food services is shown in Table 7–1. Experienced dietitians spent more time in advising, policy setting, and supervising, while the more inexperienced and entry-level dietitians were more involved in carrying out activities. The experienced dietitians also participated in a broader range of activities, including teaching, research, and marketing.[16]

In the Practice Audit conducted by the Commission on Dietetic Registration, dietitians in food service management were not singled out for study, but instead, areas of activity were reported for all those surveyed. The findings from this study were:[17]

- Both dietitians and dietetic technicians work in a variety of settings, but are concentrated in acute care, long-term care, and community settings.

Table 7-1 Average Percentage of Work Time by Categories of Food Service Activities

Category	Entry-Level RD			Beyond Entry-Level RD			Entry-Level Dietetic Technician		
	Food Service Acute	Food Service Long Term	Food Service Noninstitutional	Food Service Acute	Food Service Long Team	Food Service Noninstitutional	Food Service Acute	Food Service Long Term	Food Service Noninstitutional
Managing food service, material resources	24.3	29.0	29.8	25.6	27.0	31.1	27.9	33.9	58.3
Providing nutrition care to individuals	25.0	26.0	2.3	14.0	29.7	1.4	43.3	34.1	0.5
Providing nutrition programs for population groups	3.3	2.4	5.0	2.2	2.3	5.5	1.3	0.9	2.5
Managing financial resources	8.1	6.1	10.5	13.9	10.0	15.9	3.0	6.9	9.1
Marketing services and products	2.4	0.8	4.1	3.5	1.0	7.0	0.1	0.8	1.5
Teaching dietitians and other professionals/students	3.7	2.1	3.3	3.4	2.6	3.0	1.3	0.5	0.1
Conducting research	0.3	0.0	0.2	0.3	0.1	0.2	0.0	0.1	0.1
Managing human resources	26.8	19.9	34.6	26.0	14.6	21.2	9.7	8.0	11.3
Managing facilities	5.8	6.0	10.3	9.1	8.8	12.0	3.5	8.7	14.0
Other	0.3	7.7	0.0	2.1	3.8	2.8	10.0	6.1	2.8

Source: Reprinted with permission from *Role Delineation for Registered Dietitians and Entry-Level Dietetic Technicians,* © 1990, The American Dietetic Association.

- Both dietitians and dietetic technicians perform a variety of functions with the most common being clinical services, food services, nutrition information, and public health functions.
- The areas of activity in which dietitians and dietetic technicians are involved depend mainly on their work settings and the functions they perform.
- Levels of responsibility tend to increase with years of experience.

In the third study, a steering committee determined competencies for practice in dietetics at the entry level. They are:[18]

- Manage development and/or modification of recipes and formulas.
- Manage menu development for target populations.
- Manage production of food that meets nutrition guidelines, cost parameters, and consumer acceptance.
- Manage procurement, distribution, and service within delivery systems.
- Manage the integration of financial, human, physical, and material resources.
- Manage safety and sanitation issues related to food and nutrition.
- Supervise customer satisfaction systems for dietetic services and/or practice.
- Supervise marketing functions.
- Supervise human resource functions.
- Perform operations analysis.

STANDARDS OF PROFESSIONAL PRACTICE

Standards of professional practice have been developed by the Management in Food and Nutrition Systems Dietetic Practice Group of the ADA to describe minimum expectations in management and food service settings in evaluating quality of services, analyzing practices, and proactively developing and implementing services to maximize the nutrition, health, and well-being of clients/customers.[19] The standards are applied in five areas of practice: provision of services, application of research, communication and application of knowledge, utilization and management of resources, and quality in practice. The standards, with rationale, indicators, and examples of outcomes, are shown in their entirety in Appendix F.

CHARACTERISTICS OF SUCCESSFUL FOOD AND NUTRITION MANAGERS

Dietitians in food and nutrition management need to exhibit leadership qualities similar to those in all areas of business, health care institutions, schools, and so forth. They must manage personnel and financial resources, produce quality products and services, and communicate effectively within the organization and to the larger community. The development of "transformational leaders," defined as those who possess personal characteristics that allow them to influence the work situation, was studied by Arensberg and colleagues.[20] The transformational leader helps people and organizations function at a high level, to master change, and to plan futuristically.

Witte and Messersmith studied clinical nutrition managers and found that the training needs identified by managers were computer-assisted management, budget development, marketing, and budget management.[21]

A list of leadership competencies needed by health care food service directors is shown in Table 7–2. The competencies are typical of visionary leaders who are effective in their positions and organizations.

Table 7–2   Leadership Competencies Needed by Health Care Food Service Directors

Successful health care food service directors will:
- Exhibit astute collaborative management techniques to unify diverse points of view through consensus building, to cultivate mutually advantageous relationships in and out of the institution, and to achieve cooperation through teamwork.
- Demonstrate effective communication techniques to achieve a common understanding of personnel and departmental policies, and effective interpersonal skills through two-way communication with personnel inside and outside the department.
- Achieve an organizational structure, mission statement, policies, and procedures that effect necessary changes while managing risk taking for the department.
- Possess common-sense intelligence based on sound technological knowledge of food service, practice experience, and consideration of external business and administrative needs.
- Bear effective personnel management techniques based on sound character, compassion, insight, and personal integrity.
- Exhibit personal behaviors and attitudes consistent with professional and institutional goals.
- Demonstrate continuing pursuit of professional knowledge and growth.
- Possess effective supervisory/managerial techniques to derive optimal employee performance and appropriate documentation.
- Achieve ways to enhance performance and growth of employees.
- Possess an understanding of the politics of the institution and an ability to interface effectively with superiors.
- Exhibit effective use of resources (e.g., fiscal, personnel, materials) to facilitate planning and current operations.
- Possess analytic and decision-making techniques to achieve maximum quality for customers/clients.
- Personify behaviors and techniques that foster professional growth and leadership in department personnel.
- Demonstrate the ability to formulate a creative vision for the department that integrates mutually satisfying department and institutional goals.

Source: M. Watabe-Dawson. "Visionary Leaders Are Key to Success in Food Service." Copyright The American Dietetic Association. Reprinted by permission from *Journal of the American Dietetic Association,* vol. 95, p. 13, © 1995.

EXPANDED OPPORTUNITIES

Entry-level dietitians with management responsibilities are employed primarily in food service or clinical nutrition service operations. The predominant responsibilities at this level involve technical skills that ensure that food is procured, managed, prepared, and delivered to patients and other clients and that appropriate nutrition services are provided. With experience and perhaps advanced study, conceptual skills are utilized to identify problem areas requiring attention, to select appropriate techniques, to analyze alternative strategies, and to select solutions consistent with organization goals.

From entry-level positions, dietitians may advance to the assistant or associate director level of a department and eventually to director or chief administrator. They may manage multidepartmental units or a complex of smaller hospitals, specialty clinics, or long-term care centers. They may even become the chief operating officer of a health care facility.

Dietitians directing food and nutrition services must have a diversified multipurpose, broad-based education and experiences from which to draw for expanded roles. They must be familiar with computers, business organization, marketing, labor relations, industrial engineering, writing and media relations, public relations, financial management, data evaluation, policy formation and problem solving, decision making, negotiations, behavior modification techniques, and dealing with adaptive challenges.[22, 23]

SUMMARY

The future practitioner in food and nutrition management will have opportunities for expanded roles and responsibilities. These may include new and challenging positions not generally associated with dietetics. In the health care field, there is heightened consumer interest in what constitutes "healthy" food. The food industry wants effective marketing of their products, including information about their safety and nutrient value, and they want to develop new products. In addition, commercial food services want to meet customer demand in a financially feasible way. All these areas represent opportunities for the enterprising dietitian in an entrepreneurial way as well as within organizations.

DEFINITIONS

Food Production. The process of preparing and serving food, including purchasing, storage, and processing.

Food Services. Production and service of food; also refers to the unit or group responsible for feeding groups in an institutional setting.

Food Service Systems. Activities that together form the inputs, transformation, and outputs making up an entire food operation.

Human Resources. The personnel in an organization.

Management. Administration of the activities and functions in an organizational unit.

Quality Assurance. Certification of the continuous, optimal, effective, and efficient outcomes of a service or program.

Resource Allocation. Equitable distribution of financial, physical, and human capital.

Role Delineation Study. Study of activities and specified responsibilities of a practitioner.

Systems Approach. A process consisting of a sequence of procedures involving transformations and feedback.

Transformation. Action or activity that changes input into output in a system.

Work Processes. A sequence of actions and interactions between customers and suppliers that results in a product or service.

REFERENCES

1. Halling, J.F., and M.A. Hess. "Vision Versus Reality. ADA Members as Food/Food Management Experts." *J Am Diet Assoc* 95(1995): 169–170.

2. Cassell, J.A. *Carry the Flame: The History of the American Dietetic Association.* Chicago: The American Dietetic Association, 1990.

3. Barker, A., M. Foltz, M.B.F. Arensberg, and M.R. Schiller. *Leadership in Dietetics: Achieving a Vision for the Future.* Chicago: The American Dietetic Association, 1994.

4. Spears, M.C. *Foodservice Organization: A Managerial and Systems Approach,* 3rd ed. Englewood Cliffs, NJ: Prentice Hall, 1995.

5. Taylor, M. "Quality of Work Life Assessment of Dietitians in Business and Industry." Unpublished masters thesis. Oklahoma State University–Stillwater, 1984.

6. Liu, Y.A. "Incentives Perceived by Management Dietitians to Reduce Absenteeism Rate of Foodservice Personnel in Health Care Systems." Unpublished doctoral dissertation. Oklahoma State University–Stillwater, 1996.

7. Molt, M.K. "Dietitian's Ratings of Helpfulness of Experiences to Their Leadership Development." *National Association of College and University Food Service Journal* 19(1995): 41–50.

8. ADA. *Role Delineation for Registered Dietitians and Entry-Level Dietetic Technicians.* Chicago: The American Dietetic Association, 1990.

9. "Focus On: Dietitians Work in Correctional System." *ADA Courier* 68, no. 29(1989): 3.

10. Pilant, V.B. "Current Issues in Child Nutrition Programs." *Top Clin Nutr* 9(1994): 1–8.

11. "Position of the American Dietetic Association, Society for Nutrition Education and American School Food Service Association—Nutrition Services: An Essential Component of Comprehensive School Health Programs." *J Am Diet Assoc* 103, no. 4(2003): 505–514.

12. National Food Service Management Institute. "Job Functions and Tasks of School Nutrition Managers and District Managers/Supervisors." University of Mississippi–Oxford, 1995.

13. Jackson, R. *Nutrition and Food Services for Integrated Health Care.* Gaithersburg, MD: Aspen Publishers, 1997, p. 170.

14. Shanklin, C.W. "Opportunities in Commercial Foodservice: The Members' Perspective." *J Am Diet Assoc* 95(1995): 236–238.

15. Lechowich, K.A., and T.K. Soto. "Opportunities in Commercial Foodservice: The Industry Perspective." *J Am Diet Assoc* 95(1995): 1163–1166.

16. Kane, M.T., C.A. Estes, D.A. Colton, and C.S. Eltoft. "Role Delineation for Dietetic Practitioners: Empirical Results." *J Am Diet Assoc* 90(1990): 1124–1133.

17. Kane, M.T., A.S. Cohen, E.R. Smith, C. Lewis, and C. Leidy. "1995 Commission on Dietetic Registration Dietetics Practice Audit." *J Am Diet Assoc* 96(1996): 1292–1301.

18. Gilmore, C.J., J.O. Maillet, and B.E. Mitchell. "Determining Educational Preparation Based on Job Competencies of Entry-Level Dietetics Practitioners." *J Am Diet Assoc* 97(1997): 306–316.

19. Griffin, B., J.M. Dunn, J. Irwin, and I.F. Speranza. "Standards of Professional Practice for Dietetics Professionals in Management and Foodservice Settings." *J Am Diet Assoc* 101, no. 8(2001): 944–946.

20. Arensberg, M.B.F., M.R. Schiller, V.M. Vivian, W.A. Johnson, and S. Strasser. "Transformational Leadership of Clinical Nutrition Managers." *J Am Diet Assoc* 96(1996): 39–45.

21. Witte, S.S., and A.M. Messersmith. "Clinical Nutrition Management Practice: Responsibilities and Skill Development Strategies." *J Am Diet Assoc* 95(1995): 1113–1120.

22. Derelian, D. "President's Page: Expanded Roles Mean Expanded Opportunities." *J Am Diet Assoc* 95(1995): 708.

23. Heifetz, R.A., and D.Z. Laurie. "The Work of Leadership." *Harv Bus Rev* 75(1997): 124–134.

CHAPTER 8

Community Nutrition Practice

"Nutrition education should be an integral component of all health promotion, disease prevention, and health maintenance programs through incorporation into all appropriate nutrition communications, promotion, and education systems."[1]

Outline

- Introduction
- Community Nutrition Practice
- Public Health Nutrition
  — Prevention
  — Levels of prevention
- Activities of Community Nutritionists
- Career Paths
  — Specialty areas of practice
- Career Outlook
- Summary

INTRODUCTION

Community nutrition is the branch of nutrition that addresses the entire range of food and nutrition issues relating to individuals, families, and special groups with a common bond such as place of residence, language, culture, or health. Community nutrition programs include those that provide increased access to food resources, food and nutrition education, and health care. Public health nutrition is the component of community nutrition that is publicly funded and provided through a state or local health agency to promote health, prevent disease, and provide primary care. The community dietitian, community nutritionist, or public health nutritionist is the dietetic professional who provides nutrition services to identified groups.

Community nutrition professionals establish links with other professionals involved with the broad range of human services, including child care agencies, services to the elderly, educational institutions, and community-based research. They focus on promoting health and preventing disease in the community by using a population and systems focus and a client or personal health service approach.[2]

COMMUNITY NUTRITION PRACTICE

Community and public health nutritionists work in many settings that focus on improving the health of a population group. Positions are characterized by an emphasis on health and wellness and the application of nutrition science to maintain health. Community dietitians often work in federal, state, or local public health agency neighborhood or community health centers, industry, ambulatory care clinics, home health agencies and specialized community projects, nonprofit and for-profit private and community health agencies, institutions, private practice, and hospitals.

Each state has a department of health employing public health nutritionists. Many states also use dietitians/nutritionists in programs such as Native American health service, health and human services or welfare, department of education (school nutrition programs), and in agencies for the aging. The land-grant university in each state administers the cooperative extension program in which nutritionists, nutrition educators, and expanded food and nutrition educators are employed.

PUBLIC HEALTH NUTRITION

Practice in community nutrition is characterized by a focus on the community and includes those activities that are focused on groups rather than individuals. The largest subunit of community nutrition is the practice of public health nutrition. Whereas the practice area of community nutrition tends to be large and has a small body of defining literature, public health nutrition is well defined and includes a large body of literature discussing its role and defining characteristics. Public health nutritionists tend to work in federal, state, or local agencies.

To understand what a public health nutritionist does requires familiarity with the field of public health. Public health is defined as "the science and art of preventing disease, prolonging life, and promoting health and efficiency through organized community effort, so organizing these benefits as to enable every citizen to realize his [or her] birthright of health and longevity."[3] The public health population-based or epidemiologic approach is distinguished from the clinical or one-on-one care approach.[4] Public health focuses on the society as a whole, and the community, toward the provision of optimal health. The mission of public health is the fulfillment of society's interest in ensuring the conditions in which individuals can be healthy.[5] The goal of the discipline of public health nutrition is to promote optimal nutrition and health for all members of the population by improving nutritional status and maintaining health.[6]

A leading public health nutritionist defines a public health nutritionist as "the member of the public health agency staff who is responsible for planning, organizing, managing, directing, coordinating and evaluating the nutrition component of the health agency's services. The public health nutritionist establishes linkages with related community nutrition programs, nutrition education, food assistance, social or welfare services, care services to the elderly, other human services and community-based research."[7]

The public health approach has the following distinguishing characteristics:

- Uses interventions that promote health and prevent communicable or chronic diseases by managing or controlling the community environment
- Promotes a healthy lifestyle as a shared value for all people
- Directs money and energy to the problems that affect the lives of the largest number of people in the community
- Targets the unserved or underserved by virtue of income, age, ethnicity, heredity, or lifestyle who are vulnerable to disease, hunger, or malnutrition
- Requires the collaboration of the public, consumers, community leaders, legislators, policy makers, administrators, and health and human service professionals in assessing and responding to community needs and consumer demands
- Monitors the health of the people in the community to ensure that the public health system achieves its objectives and responds to needs

Prevention

The prevention of illness is the primary purpose of public health. Prevention may take place at any point along the spectrum from prevention of disease to the prevention of impairment or disability. Prevention has three essential components: (1) personal health, (2) community based, and (3) social policies/systems based. Each component has distinct roles, importance, and focus. Community nutrition practice involves making appropriate and coordinated use of each. Personal health deals with prevention issues at the individual level, such as working with a client to improve the diet for health promotion purposes. Community-based prevention is targeted toward groups such as the Five-a-Day campaign that focuses on increased consumption of fruits and vegetables or campaigns that focus on weight loss. Social policies/systems-level prevention focuses on changing policies and law so that the goals of prevention practice are achieved (e.g., laws regarding food safety, tobacco, or alcohol).

Levels of Prevention

For each of the three components of prevention, there are three levels of prevention. *Primary prevention* or health promotion efforts involves prevention of the disease itself and serves to maintain a state of wellness. *Secondary prevention* is the detection, diagnosis, and intervention early in the disease process to minimize disabling effects. *Tertiary prevention* is directed at treating and rehabilitating persons with diagnosed health conditions to prevent or delay their disability, pain, suffering, and premature death.[8]

ACTIVITIES OF COMMUNITY NUTRITIONISTS

About 11 percent of RDs and 10 percent of DTRs work in community nutrition.[9] Five percent of the RDs and 7 percent of the DTRs work in the Women's, Infants, and Children's (WIC) programs. WIC provides supplemental food and nutrition education and works to provide access to health services for low-income pregnant, breastfeeding, and nonbreastfeeding women and their children up to 5 years of age. Other positions include maternal and child nutrition, adult health, food service management, and children with special health care needs.[10]

For individuals to benefit from nutrition research, nutritionists working in the community must be able to translate science into practical dietary guidance. In useful terms, this means providing information about foods that are affordable and available in local markets. All nutritionists must be experts in normal and clinical nutrition and be competent in bringing about changes in eating behavior. To be a credible nutrition resource, the RD who works in public health nutrition must understand the fundamentals of nutrition, food science, and dietetics, as well as have an underlying knowledge of human physiology, chemistry, biochemistry, and behavioral sciences. This includes an in-depth knowledge of nutritional needs during all stages of the life span because people of all ages will be served in the various programs. Awareness of family-centered care and case management is important as is the ability to function as a clinical or public health team member for diagnostic, evaluative, and follow-up programs that provide services for clients in a comprehensive, culturally sensitive, and community-based service system.[11] The nutritionist must develop political and communication skills and be knowledgeable about public policy development and strategic planning.[12–14]

Some nutritionists focus primarily on population-based interventions for health promotion and disease prevention. Others who provide more direct nutrition care usually focus their energies on providing nutrition services to medically high-risk persons. There are, however, many nutritionists whose positions are a mix of functions that include community assessment and program development along with client-focused clinical care.

The dietitian's duties may include nutrition training for other agency staff as well as providing technical assistance to other professionals; serving as a resource to the public, media, business, and industry; and advocating for needed nutrition policy at the local, state, and/or federal level. Others may include advising the agency administrator, policy makers, and staff on current nutrition research findings that can contribute to the public's health and to the organization's mission, policies, and programs.

CAREER PATHS

The term *public health nutritionist* has usually been reserved for the member of the nutrition team who has a master's degree in public health nutrition. This training includes skills required to participate in policy analysis and program development. The public health nutritionist knows the practical aspects of assessing nutritional needs of a community and develops skills in planning, evaluating, and implementing programs to meet these needs. Academic training includes a knowledge of biostatistics and a skill in collecting, compiling, analyzing, and reporting demographic, health, and food consumption data as well as an understanding of the epidemiology of health and disease distribution patterns in the population and studying trends over time. According to Dodds and Kaufman, public health nutrition personnel can be placed in three major classes based on their responsibilities: management, professional, or technical.[15] These series are shown in Table 8–1.

Table 8–1 Positions of Public Health Nutritionists

Class	Title of Position	Functions
Management	Public health director Assistant public health director	Policy making, planning, management, supervision, fiscal control
Professional	Public health nutrition consultant Public health nutritionist Clinical nutritionist Nutritionist	Planning and evaluation, consultation, care coordination, case management, counseling
Technical	Nutrition technician Nutrition assistant	Education, screening, recordkeeping, outreach

Source: Adapted with permission from J.M. Dodds and M. Kaufman, *Personnel in Public Health Nutrition for the 1990s. A Comprehensive Guide.* Washington, DC: The Public Foundation, 1991.

Specialty Areas of Practice

Several career paths are available to the public health nutritionist in areas considered "specialties." Typical of these are the following: *Adult health promotion/ chronic disease prevention and control specialists* may work in health care facilities, worksite health promotion, and community health agencies. Knowledge of nutritional management of specific chronic diseases and behavioral and lifestyle change methodologies is required.

Specialists working with special health care needs related to developmental diseases and chronic disabling conditions need clinical knowledge of child growth and development with an emphasis on the effects of mental retardation, developmental disabilities, and rehabilitation. Knowledge of techniques of feeding under special conditions is also required.

Maternal and child health specialists understand principles of nutrition in pregnancy and lactation and in infancy, childhood, and adolescence. This includes the physical, psychological, and socioeconomic aspects of these early periods of life.

Communication and media specialists must have knowledge of how individuals learn and of nutrition education methodology. They must also know how to use media effectively to design and implement nutrition promotion campaigns through a variety of communication channels, including television, radio, newspapers, magazines, and computers in various settings.

Data management and nutrition surveillance nutritionists require additional training in biostatistics, epidemiology, and computer-based data management. Their responsibilities include the development of user-friendly systems for collecting, analyzing, interpreting, and presenting numerical data to be used in community program planning.

Environmental health and food safety specialists have advanced knowledge and skills in food science, food processing technology, microbiology, epidemiology, and food safety laws and regulations. They must be able to interpret federal, state, and local regulations regarding food safety.

Food service systems management for health care and group care facilities specialists have an in-depth knowledge of food service systems management, health care financing, clinical nutrition, and nutritional care planning.

Home health specialists have advanced knowledge of diet therapy for chronic disease and chronic disabling conditions of adults and children.

Research specialists need to know how to prepare grant proposals, manage data, coordinate field-based studies, and design research protocols.

Educators of public health nutrition professionals must have the knowledge and skills to prepare students for practice in public health or community health.

CAREER OUTLOOK

Community nutrition practice is changing as the overall health care system evolves. Expanding opportunities during a time of decreased funding requires dietitians working in the community to be well prepared academically to compete. At the same time, more nutrition personnel with advanced clinical skills are needed to provide intensive nutritional care in the home and community to medically high-risk pregnant women, disabled and chronically ill infants and children, chronically ill adults, and the elderly.

Public health agencies are expected to assume additional population-focused responsibilities, and nutrition professionals will likely shift from a client-focused system with direct care service responsibilities to a population/systems focus with more administrative and planning-related functions.[16] Some in public health will continue to provide personal health services, particularly in areas where providers are limited or where certain high-risk populations are underserved. This shift from a client to a population focus will occur at different rates. In communities where access to clinical, prevention, and therapeutic services is limited, the transition will be slow. Public health and community nutrition professionals will need to be proactive and creative in assuming their responsibilities.[17]

SUMMARY

Community nutrition is an area in which professionals interact with community groups and individuals to promote health and prevent disease. Dietitians/nutritionists working in community nutrition hold positions in areas of public health, programs for the aging, cooperative extension, outpatient and public health clinics, state and local government, and agencies dealing with chronic disease. The emphasis is on meeting the nutritional needs of persons during all stages of life, thus maintaining health and preventing disease.

DEFINITIONS

Client. The recipient of services or products.

Client-Based Focus. Use of assessment and diagnostic methods to identify individuals at high medical and/or nutrition risk and provide interventions in the form of one-on-one counseling or small group counseling and education as part of a clinic or health care.

Community. Group of persons whose members share a common bond such as living in the same geographic area or sharing the same culture or language.

Community Assessment. Formal process of collecting and evaluating relevant information about the ecology of a particular community and applying the data to determine met and unmet needs of the community.

Community Health Services. Health services provided for a specific group of people who have a common bond such as language, geographic area, socioeconomic needs, or similar health problems.

Health Care Team. A group of health professionals who work together with the common objective of providing comprehensive and coordinated health care services to individuals and their families.

Health Promotion/Disease Prevention. Education and preventive health measures directed toward basically healthy populations to foster wellness and prevent illness.

Nutrition Assessment. Evaluation of an individual's nutritional status based on anthropometric, biochemical, clinical, and dietary information.

Population-Based Focus. Epidemiologic methods to describe health and nutrition needs in the community and serve as the basis for designing interventions to reach the general population or large segments of the population at particular risk.

Program Planning. The process by which administrators assess needs and develop a plan to meet these needs.

REFERENCES

1. ADA. "Position of the American Dietetic Association: Nutrition Education for the Public." *J Am Diet Assoc* 96(1996): 1183–1187.

2. Public Health Nutrition Practice Group of the American Dietetic Association. "Guidelines for Community Nutrition Supervised Practice Experience." Chicago: The American Dietetic Association, 1995.

3. Winslow, C.E.A. "The Untitled Field of Public Health." *Mod Med* 2(1920): 183.

4. Kaufman, M. *Nutrition in Public Health: A Handbook for Developing Programs and Services*. Rockville, MD: Aspen Publishers, 1990.

5. Institute of Medicine. *The Future of Public Health*. Washington, DC: National Academy Press, 1988.

6. *Strategies for Success: Curriculum Guide for Graduate Programs in Public Health Nutrition*. Washington, DC: Association of the Faculties of Graduate Programs in Public Health Nutrition, 1990.

7. See Note 4.

8. Ibid.

9. Rogers, D. "Report on the ADA 2002 Dietetics Compensation and Benefits Survey." *J Am Diet Assoc* 103, no. 2(2003): 243–255.

10. "ASTPHND Biennial Profile of Personnel in Public Health Nutrition." Recruitment of Public/Community Nutritionist workshop. Association of State and Territorial Public Health Nutrition Directors, 1994.

11. See Note 4.

12. *Strategies for Success: Curriculum Guide for Graduate Programs in Public Health Nutrition*. Washington, DC: Association of the Faculties of Graduate Programs in Public Health Nutrition, 1990.

13. Dodds, J.M., and M. Kaufman. *Personnel in Public Health Nutrition for the 1990s: A Comprehensive Guide*. Washington, DC: The Public Health Foundation, 1991.

14. ASPH. *Graduate Education for Public Health*. Washington, DC: Association of Schools of Public Health, 1988.

15. Dodds, J.M., and M. Kaufman. *Personnel in Public Health Nutrition for the 1990s: A Comprehensive Guide*. Washington, DC: The Public Health Foundation, 1991.

16. Story, M., B. Haughton, and M. Olmstead-Schafer. "Future Training Needs in Public Health Nutrition. Results of a National Delphi Survey." Unpublished manuscript.

17. Ibid.

CHAPTER 9

The Consultant in Health Care, Business, and Private Practice

"Many dietitians are doing what has not been done before. They embody the entrepreneurial spirit, their ingenuity, creative verve, and aggressiveness are leading them and the dietetics profession into new fields of experience."[1]

Outline

- Introduction
- Establishing a Practice
  — Contracts and fees
- The Consultant in Health Care and Extended Care
  — Regulations
  — Areas of practice
  — Roles and responsibilities
  — Standards for quality assurance
- The Consultant in Business Practice
  — Practice qualifications
  — Areas of practice
- The Dietitian in Private Practice
  — Entering a practice
  — Marketing
  — Areas of practice
  — Practice roles
  — ADA network providers
- Ethical and Legal Bases of Practice
- Summary

INTRODUCTION

In the 2002 Dietitian Compensation and Benefits Survey, it was reported that 11 percent of RDs and about 2 percent of DTRs indicated their primary practice area was in consultation and business. About 3 percent of the RDs work in private practice.[2] Many dietitians have found that self-employment with the flexibility of times as well as hours of work and compensation is an attractive alternative to more traditional positions. An entrepreneurial drive is often the impetus for professionals to become consultants or to establish their own practice although many do so because of family or other obligations.

Health care institutions have, for the past several years, moved an increasing number of services away from inpatient care into outpatient clinics and other community agencies as well as the home. Governmental regulations have led further to the need for nutrition consultants in extended care facilities, and both these trends have led to the need for a greater number of persons as consultants rather than as full-time employees.

Three types of consultant practice are discussed in this chapter: consultants in health care and extended care; consultation in business practice; and dietitians in private practice.

ESTABLISHING A PRACTICE

Starting a practice as a consultant or in private practice requires thought and planning. Two excellent publications that are available to guide the dietitian in planning are Helm's *The Competitive Edge* (1995) and Helm's *The Entrepreneurial Nutritionist* (1991).[3,4] A self-assessment is the first step. Personal characteristics are important because an individual needs to be self-directed, energetic, and action oriented. A list of questions that can be used to determine an individual's readiness to enter private practice is shown in Table 9–1.

When the decision has been made to start a consulting practice, several actions need to be taken. If an office is established, appropriate office equipment must be obtained and decisions made about secretarial and/or office manager assistance. Networking with other successful dietitians through one or more practice groups is an excellent way of gaining valuable start-up information. Mentors may be found and networks established from these contacts. Guides to legal and other practical considerations are provided by reading Cross's 1995 article.[5] Professional liability insurance must be considered early in the planning stages. This insurance is available through the American Dietetic Association (ADA).

The consultant often locates "accounts" or positions though networking. Initiating contacts with facilities followed by interviews with the administrator and meeting other key personnel should occur. Negotiations should include a clear

Table 9–1   Questionnaire to Determine Readiness for Private Practice

Are you a self-starter?
3—I do things on my own—nobody has to tell me what or when to get going.
2—If someone gets me started, I keep going by myself.
1—Easy does it! Keep prodding me and I will move along fine.

Are you a risk taker?
3—I'll take a chance, even if I am unsure of success.
2—I'll jump in, if I am fairly sure of succeeding.
1—Uncertainty is not for me—I'll wait until success is guaranteed.

Do you have a positive, friendly interest in others?
3—I enjoy new people and can get along with just about anybody.
2—I am most comfortable with existing friends and don't need anyone else.
1—Meeting new people is not my forte. I prefer being alone.

Are you a leader?
3—I can get most people to go along when I start something.
2—I can give the orders if someone else tells me what we should do.
1—I let someone else get things moving. Then I go along if I feel like it.

Can you handle responsibility?
3—I like to take charge of things and see them through.
2—I'll take over if I have to, but I'd rather let someone else be responsible.
1—I would just rather not have the final responsibility.

Are you a good organizer?
3—I like to make plans and check them off. I'm usually the one to get things lined up when the group wants to do something.
2—I do all right until things get too confused. Then I quit.
1—Things get done as they come. I don't like too much structure.

Are you prepared to put in long hours?
3—I can keep going long and hard for something I want.
2—I'll work hard for a while, but when I've had enough, that's it.
1—It will either happen or it won't, so there is no merit in working yourself to death.

Do you make up your mind quickly?
3—If I have to, I can make up my mind in a hurry and it usually turns out okay.
2—I need time to decide. When I make up my mind too fast, I often think later I should have decided the other way.
1—I simply can't decide without considering all the details and discussing them with others.

Can people rely on you?
3—I say what I mean and I deliver. It's simplest.
2—I try to be on the level, but sometimes I don't know or can't deliver but don't really want to admit it.
1—People never really pay attention, so I just say whatever is easiest.

(continues)

Table 9–1   continued

Can you withstand reversals without quitting?
3—Once I've made up my mind, nothing stops me.
2—I usually finish what I start—if it goes well.
1—If it doesn't go right away, I see no reason to keep hammering away.

Total your score. If your score is 24–30, you probably have what it takes to be in private practice in nutrition. If your score is 17–23, running a business of your own would likely be an uphill battle. A total score below 16 suggests that you may not be ready to be independent in business. Rare is the person who has an abundance of all the traits essential to business success or who does not need to improve in one or more areas to be better in business. There are ways to strengthen them both before and after you begin your business. Attend conferences and lectures of aspects of private practice in nutrition and on business operations in general. Experts on business management often have tips gathered through years of experience. Read books and articles to keep up with developments in the field of nutrition and in the business world.

Source: A.T. Cross, "Practical and Legal Considerations of Private Nutrition Practice," *J Am Diet Assoc* 95(1995): 21–29.

understanding of the amount of time the consultant will be needed. Although regulations in a health care facility may require only a minimum number of hours per month, there may be compelling reasons for more time to be spent in the facility. For instance, in larger institutions with a large number of residents or institutions in which a number of residents require skilled care, additional time will be needed by the consultant.

The dietitian establishing a private practice needs the services of at least three professionals: a lawyer, an accountant, and a banker.[6] They will guide the dietitian in many business decisions that he or she may not have the skills or expertise to make alone. Success in private practice depends on the individual's personal characteristics for business ownership, the type of legal and financial ownership structure under which the business operates, the adequacy of start-up funding, and the appropriate pricing of services.[7]

Depending on the consultant's business organization—partnership, corporation, sole practitioner, and so forth—the consultant may have mentors and partners and also a board of directors. If so, the organization's lawyer, banker, and accountant should serve on the board. Most cities have a small business association or an economic development center, both of which provide assistance to persons in the early stages of establishing a business or practice. Banks and investment companies often provide advice and assistance to entrepreneurs starting a business and may provide services specifically for women.

Contracts and Fees

A major consideration for the dietitian in consultation and private practice is setting prices and fees and obtaining reimbursement for services. A contract that specifies the services to be provided, the amount of time alloted the services, and fees to be assessed is the first step. Establishing and negotiating the ground rules are important in the initial stages of the process.[8]

The consultant in health care facilities can gain information about rates by looking at pay levels in the area and region for different types of consulting work and for basic salary levels.

Expenses such as liability insurance, mileage and travel expenses, and any educational components needed should be added to arrive at a fee. A helpful discussion on the process of setting fees is presented in *The Entrepreneurial Nutritionist*.[9]

Dietitians who receive reimbursement from insurers or complementary networks or medical nutrition therapy (MNT) will also be involved in negotiating fees. The use of MNT codes is used in establishing payment rates in private practice.[10]

THE CONSULTANT IN HEALTH CARE
AND EXTENDED CARE

The role of the consultant in health care facilities and extended care became important with the enactment of the Medicare regulations by the Health Care Financing Administration in the 1960s. Long-term care facilities (primarily nursing homes) were required to hire a qualified dietitian, and the demand for consultant dietitians rapidly increased as a result. From a limited employment area with little history, few guidelines, and dietitians "on their own" insofar as job requirements and benefits were concerned, consultation in health care facilities became one in which many dietitians soon found positions. Many had been out of the workforce for periods of time but returned to practice with these opportunities. Some of the dietitians needed to be updated in practice knowledge and skills and turned to continuing education opportunities to gain the necessary information to practice as a consultant. By 1975, 90 percent of skilled nursing homes used the services of a dietitian.[11]

The amount of time a dietitian is needed is not specified in federal regulations. Instead, they state that the consultant's visits should be of "sufficient frequency to meet the food and nutrition needs of the facility."[12] State licensing requirements, however, frequently specify a minimum of 8 hours a month. A dietitian contracts with a facility for the amount of time needed, at or above the minimum, to meet the facility's needs.

Most consultants are employed on a part-time basis in one or more facilities, although the individual's time commitment could be full time, depending on the number of facilities in which the consultant works and the amount of time he or she chooses to work. Some dietitians are employed full time for a multifacility chain or in one large facility.

Regulations

A consultant dietitian must be familiar with state and federal regulations that apply to long-term/extended care facilities. The health department in each state can provide copies of both the state and federal regulations. Federal regulations are precise concerning both the physical plant and the operation and staffing of the facility. In general, state regulations follow the federal but may be even more specific in certain areas. Each facility has its own procedures and set of regulations governing its operation. The consultant needs to be thoroughly familiar with these as well as the policies and goals of the facility.

The Omnibus Reconciliation Act of 1987 (updated in 1991) published regulations for long-term care that are followed in nursing homes and other facilities receiving federal Medicare funds.[13] The effect of Medicare regulations in dietetic practice was discussed by Johnson and Coulston[14] in relation to reimbursement for nutrition care. Many long-term care facilities seek accreditation from the Joint Commission on Accreditation of Healthcare Organizations, which also sets specific regulations for care.[15]

Areas of Practice

Long-term care facilities include nursing homes, skilled nursing facilities, subacute centers, adult day care, residential care facilities, and alcohol and drug rehabilitation facilities. Long-term care facilities may be privately owned, city or county owned, owned by religious organizations, or owned by corporations. They may be for-profit or not-for-profit and may range in size from 50 to 200 beds or more.

Consultants may also be hired to visit developmentally disabled clients in their homes. In addition, some state health departments contract with consultants to provide services for Women, Infants, and Children program participants. Other consultants work in home health care, congregate feeding sites, senior citizen centers, correctional facilities, group homes for the developmentally disabled, hospice programs, and small rural hospitals.

Roles and Responsibilities

A consultant functions primarily in an advisory capacity within a facility; however, he or she has ethical and professional responsibilities for the nutritional care of the residents. By developing rapport and using organizational skills, the consultant is able to accomplish the needed tasks. Because he or she is usually not in the facility full time, the day-to-day supervision may be provided by a dietetic manager or technician.

When a consultant begins employment in a facility, one of the first activities should be an assessment of needs in food service and nutrition services for the residents to use as a guide for further planning and action. Documentation of observations and plans for future visits is very important, beginning with the first visit. The typical activities a consultant performs during a visit to the facility may include the following:[16]

- Conferring with the dietary manager and the administrator about day-to-day operations and any problems that need to be addressed during the visit
- Performing nutrition assessments of new residents and conducting a follow-up for all others
- Checking at-risk residents and making recommendations for further nutritional care as indicated. This includes noting unexplained changes in weight or the development of pressure ulcers, checking those on tube feedings, and noting signs of dehydration or otherwise poor nutritional status[17–19]
- Observing the meal service and eating a meal to evaluate food quality
- Making nutrition rounds at meal time to observe the residents' acceptance of the food and their food intakes
- Conducting educational in-service sessions for employees and exchanging information regarding departmental activities
- Documenting all activities with any recommendations for follow-up

The consultant may be responsible for developing policy and procedure manuals for the quality improvement program, for safety and sanitation procedures, or for budget management.[20] The reference diet manual should be reviewed and signed by the chief of the medical staff at least annually and should be updated regularly.

Consultants may also teach dietetic technician students and conduct classes for dietary managers. They may serve as preceptors for students in supervised experiences in long-term care.

Standards for Quality Assurance

The Consultant Dietitian-Health Care Facilities practice group has developed standards of practice for consultant dietitians in health care facilities as a guide for quality assurance. The standards specify six general areas of activity with examples of outcomes. They include provision of services, application of research, communication and application of knowledge, utilization and management of resources, and continued competence and professional accountability.[21] The full text is found in Appendix F.

Through written documentation, consultant dietitians can verify actual performance and implement action to meet the expected criteria. The standards also help dietitians develop a workable plan to meet the responsibilities for which they have contracted and to evaluate their own knowledge, clinical experience, and management expertise.

Consultant practice has expanded over the years. For example, settings where consultant dietitians now work include special dementia units, assisted living, psychiatric facilities for the developmentally disabled and mentally retarded, and correctional facilities. Home care, adult day care, group homes, and retirement communities are further areas of opportunity for the consultant dietitian in health care.

THE CONSULTANT IN BUSINESS PRACTICE

Only imagination and personal ambition might limit the opportunities for experienced dietitians to be employed in business practice. Potential practice areas as identified by the Nutrition Entrepreneurs practice group of the ADA include service for individuals, corporations, the media, restaurants, food companies, and sports or health facilities. Another practice group, the Dietitians in Business and Communication, identify their members as presidents, vice presidents, food service directors, food stylists, researchers, consultants, sales managers, marketing managers, restaurateurs, test kitchen managers, and software specialists.

In the early 1990s, through its strategic planning activities, the ADA identified commercial food service as a major market linkage for dietetic services. It was pointed out that to compete in this environment, management of rapid product introduction and of sales among a variety of food products and knowledge of rapidly changing technology and environmental controls are essential.[22]

What is unique about the dietitian working as a consultant in business practice? Dietitians who decide to enter a business consulting practice are risk takers. They like to take on new challenges and to become part of a powerful group of innovative thinkers and doers. They are energetic and versatile professionals with a wide range of interests and agendas in the business community. They are dietitians in leadership positions among many who have chosen nontraditional career paths.

Although many of the responsibilities for a consultant may be similar to those of a full-time dietitian, one of the main differences is in the duration of the assignment. The consultant in business practice is given a short-term contract with an identified scope. The scope of services is usually an assignment to set up or improve the business practice of the client. It may also be a specific project with a defined beginning and end time period. Examples of activities the consultant may perform include evaluating staffing patterns, establishing an inventory and cost control system, planning a new production or service system, and recommending equipment purchases.

Practice Qualifications

The opportunities for the entry-level dietitian to work as a consultant in business practices are limited because of the depth of knowledge and experience needed to be successful as a consultant. Older students who have life experiences or expertise in another profession have an advantage in this area of practice. Another feature of business consultation is that most dietitians are sole operators. Many do not employ full-time secretarial staff or other assistants. If they have an overload of work or need the services of other experts to complete an assignment, they may contract out portions of jobs while still maintaining overall control.

Areas of Practice

A limited number of business consulting firms do employ entry-level dietitians for consulting but in a defined scope of responsibility. The usual requirement is that the dietitian is experienced in some area (e.g., as a clinical dietitian in a health care facility or manager of a food service system). The dietitian may also have worked as an assistant to another dietitian for a food processor, equipment manufacturer, publisher, marketing company, or software specialist. When hired, he or she may first be assigned to a team leader to work on a specific part of a major project. With experience, there may be opportunities to expand into other nontraditional roles such as facility management, accounting, design, sales, or marketing. The range of expanded responsibility is dependent on the scope of the services performed by the company and those that the dietitian can develop for the company.

The following guidelines have been proposed for those who may be thinking of moving into management with the goal of consultation or his or her own business:[23]

- Discuss new plans with the immediate supervisor
- Seek advice from a veteran manager or mentor
- React deliberately rather than spontaneously
- Weigh solutions against the mission of the organization
- Practice active listening with everyone involved
- Investigate the literature for continued information and self-education

THE DIETITIAN IN PRIVATE PRACTICE

Many dietitians today become entrepreneurs and enter private practice for a variety of reasons. Some seek new and innovative opportunities out of choice; others do so due to circumstances that make private practice a viable option. Examples of the latter might be the loss of a job or the need to work varying hours because of family responsibilities. Opportunities for women in the business world are unquestionably increasing. The health care industry continues to downsize from large centralized centers to outpatient and community centers with fewer staff. Many dietitians seek greater independence and new challenges and, along with a business climate that encourages entrepreneurs, find satisfying careers in private practice.[24]

Not all entrepreneurs start a business as such. Some work at home and may combine home and family responsibilities with part-time, contract-type work including consulting, writing, computer searches, home visits, and so forth. Others may open an office, hire assistants, and establish a full-time practice or business.[25]

Entering a Practice

The dietitian who enters private practice needs to exhibit certain personal characteristics including determination, initiative, and perseverance.[26] The questions shown in Table 9–1 are especially important for the dietitian in private practice to assess readiness to practice.

Marketing

In whatever area of private practice a dietitian pursues, marketing is an essential part of the planning. To gain the "competitive edge," clients and the public will be most receptive when they are convinced that the service or product being offered is one they trust and need. Establishing credibility and visibility is therefore a large part of a successful marketing strategy. It is often more difficult to market a service than a product; however, the marketing process is facilitated by the creation of an image and a message that establishes the most positive aspects of the service to be provided. Dietitians have an advantage in offering dietetic services in that improved or optimal health is the outcome.

Many successful entrepreneurial dietitians are in nontraditional careers, creating opportunities for themselves and others where none existed before. This is perhaps why private practice is an increasingly attractive option for many dietitians.

Areas of Practice

The consultant in private practice will usually be located outside an organization but may also be an "intrapreneur" or one within an organization who develops new ideas or services that are used profitably in some way. The work setting is as diverse as the practitioner's interests and expertise as well as the market demands.[27,28] This is illustrated in Table 9–2.

The professional services provided are influenced by the needs of the consumer,[29] the demands and changing environments of health care,[30] changes in regulatory agencies, increased autonomy, and advances in science and technology.[31] As new ideas are disseminated and needs identified, more roles are defined for the private practitioner. Dietitians may form alliances and networks to provide services. By teaming with other professionals, the ability to market services and products and share business expense is enhanced. The opportunities through a wider range of contacts may also be increased. Examples of such associations are preferred provider organizations to managed care companies, dietitian networks, or

Table 9–2 Settings for Consulting in Private Practice

Private office
Private home
Physician or other allied health professional offices
Home health care
Health/fitness centers and spas
Community-based programs
Schools
Hospitals
Day homes
Senior citizen centers
Nursing homes
Contracts with government agencies
Media and communications
Grocery stores
Restaurant and culinary industry (chefs)
Corporate settings or worksites
Business and industry
Food companies
Hotels and resorts
Research centers
Medical education consulting firms
Private specialty clinics (sports medicine clinics, eating disorder clinics, diabetes, renal, oncology, HIV/AIDS)
Rehabilitation centers

Source: Alexander-Israel, D., and C. Roman-Shriver, In: *Dietetics: Practice and Future Trends.* E.A. Winterfeldt, M.L. Bogle, and L.L. Ebro. Aspen Publishers, Gaithersburg, MD, 1998, p. 208.

dietitian independent practice associations.[32] DPGs in the ADA also provide a way for networking to occur among professionals.

Practice Roles

Consultants in private practice may teach clients and consumers in areas ranging from wellness and prevention; to medical nutrition therapy, business and industry, education and training, food service and culinary trades; and writing and media presentation. A list of activities is shown in Table 9–3 as examples of the types of services that consultants may perform.

Table 9–3   Roles of Consultants in Private Practice

Assessment of nutritional status
Menu evaluation and planning
Recipe evaluation and modification
One-on-one counseling
Family counseling
Group education
Monitoring of nutritional intervention
Dietary analysis and evaluation of products
Consultant to agencies, institutions, and programs with nutritional components (extended care, school food service, hospital, government agencies, clinics)
Consultant to professionals (health care, food service, culinary industry)
Consultant to corporations (fitness centers, wellness/health promotion programs, benefits departments)
Writing for the lay public (books, newsletters, magazines, and newspaper articles)
Professional publications
Group training, presentations, workshops
Developing nutritious/healthier menu items for restaurants
Restaurant and culinary staff training
Assistance in marketing nutrition in restaurants
Computer/software programming (total quality management, nutrition education, food service, clinical nutrition)
Developing and marketing nutrition education programs (private and public markets)
Supermarket tours and grocery information guides
Nutrition labeling information
Rehabilitation and sports injury consultation
Nutrition care planning
Monitoring compliance with local, state, federal regulations (long-term care facilities, drug-alcohol centers, prisons)
Developing, administering, evaluating nutrition standards
Multidisciplinary preventive and therapeutic services

Source: Alexander-Israel, D., C. Roman-Shriver, In: *Dietetics: Practice and Future Trends.* E.A. Winterfeldt, M.L. Bogle, and L.L. Ebro. Aspen Publishers, Gaithersburg, MD, 1998, p. 209.

Practice roles can often be expanded with more training in business, marketing, and communications and with the development of new skills that cross the boundaries of other health professionals.[33] For example, dietitians can become proficient at taking blood pressures and body composition measurements in the home care setting; can secure American College of Sports Medicine Exercise Test Technology Certification for performing electrocardiogram-monitored stress tests in sports medicine clinics; Clinical Laboratory Improvement Certification for blood analysis; or can use phlebotomy skills in wellness programs.

Emerging roles demand expanding the dietitian's scope of practice and skills and capitalizing on the talents that are unique to dietitians.[34] Among these are the ability to apply food and nutrition knowledge, use nutrition assessment tools, apply lifestyle-change education to prevent or manage disease, and to collect data on positive outcomes of nutrition intervention in quality of life and reduced overall health care costs.

ADA Network Providers

The nationwide nutrition network is a service offered by the ADA whereby requests for nutrition counseling may be referred to dietitian-subscribers to the service. The service includes business-related dietetic practice and marketing to business and industry.[35]

ETHICAL AND LEGAL BASES OF PRACTICE

Important guides for the dietitian are the professional code of conduct (Appendix A) and any applicable rule or statute of practice from the state and local authorities under whose jurisdiction the dietitian practices. These documents will clarify disciplinary action that can be taken by the professional or regulatory agencies on violations of the code covering such activities as advertising and practicing medicine versus nutrition. When establishing a business, the advice of an attorney is indispensable relative to business law and limits on the private practice of nutrition and the laws of the state in which the practice is established.

SUMMARY

Traditional institutional roles for dietitians, especially in clinical dietetics, are still predominant practice settings; however, many dietitians are using their clinical background to become entrepreneurs in their own practice. The dietitian who possesses the needed personal attributes plus the initiative and creativity needed for entrepreneurial success may find a rewarding new career in consultation in health care facilities, in business, or in private practice.

DEFINITIONS

Client. The recipient of services or products.

Consultant. A skilled or knowledgeable person qualified to give expert professional advice.

Continuous Quality Improvement. The continued study and improvement of the process and outcomes of health care services to meet the needs of those served. Specific structured problem-solving methods are used that rely on data and group process tools.

Intrapreneur. A person within an organization who develops new ideas or services, usually for a profit.

Joint Commission on Accreditation of Healthcare Organizations (The Joint Commission). The accrediting agency that sets standards for health care units and conducts reviews based on the standards for those institutions requesting the accreditation. The standards are identified as essential factors that result in safe, effective, high-yield patient care.

Long-Term Care. Assistance provided over time to people with chronic health conditions and/or physical disabilities and those who are unable to care for themselves.

Managed Care. A system of health care administered by an entity outside a hospital or health care institution in which access, cost, and quality of care are controlled by direct intervention before or during service for purposes of creating efficiencies and/or reducing costs.

Medicare. The federal insurance program that provides hospital and medical services for individuals 65 years of age or older, individuals of any age who have permanent kidney failure that requires dialysis or a kidney replacement, and certain individuals younger than 65 years of age who have disabilities.

Nutrition Assessment. Evaluation of an individual's nutritional status based on anthropometric, biochemical, clinical, and dietary information.

Nutrition Screening. The use of diagnostic methodology to determine nutritional risk and the necessity of an in-depth nutrition assessment.

Omnibus Budget Reconciliation Act (OBRA). Legislation that led to regulations for residents in long-term care facilities. The regulations are developed and implemented by the Centers for Medicare and Medicaid Services.

Private Practice. Self-employment in which a person manages his or her own working career.

Subacute Care. Services provided in a treatment unit, usually after acute hospital care and before home care or a long-term care facility.

REFERENCES

1. Helm, K.K. *The Entrepreneurial Nutritionist,* 2nd ed. Lake Dallas, TX: K.K. Helm Publications, 1991.
2. Rogers, D. "Report on the ADA 2002 Dietetics Compensation Benefits Survey." *J Am Diet Assoc* 103, no. 2(2003): 243–255.
3. Helm, K.K. *The Competitive Edge: Advanced Marketing for Dietetic Professionals.* Chicago: The American Dietetic Association, 1995.
4. See Note 1.
5. Cross, A.T. "Practical and Legal Considerations of Private Nutrition Practice." *J Am Diet Assoc* 95(1995): 21–29.
6. Norton, L.C. "The Consultant in Business Practice. In *Dietetics: Practice and Future Trends,* E.A. Winterfeldt, M.L. Bogle, and L.L. Ebro, eds. Gaithersburg, MD: Aspen Publishers, 1998, p. 236.
7. See Note 5.
8. McCafree, J. "Contract Basics: What a Dietitian Should Know." *J Am Diet Assoc* 103, no. 4(2003): 429–430.
9. See Note 1.
10. Albardo, M. "Understanding and Negotiating Access Contracts with Insurers and Complementary Networks." *J Am Diet Assoc* 102, no. 2(2002): 187–189; and Myers, E.F., P. Michael, and K.C. Duester. "Tips for Contract Negotiations and Establishing MNT Rates." *J Am Diet Assoc* 101, no. 6(2001): 624–626.
11. Office of Nursing Home Affairs. *Long-Term Care Improvement Study.* DHEW Publication No. C05.76-50021, 1975.
12. "Skilled Nursing Facilities: Standards for Certification and Participation in Medicare and Medicaid Programs." *Federal Register* 39(January 17, 1974): 22–38.
13. Robinson, G., and C. Russell. "OBRA Regulations Revisited." *Diet Curric* 23(1996): 15–20.
14. Johnson, R.K., and A.M. Coulston. "Medicare: Reimbursement Rules, Impediments, and Opportunities for Dietitians." *J Am Diet Assoc* 95(1995): 1378–1380.
15. Robinson, G.E. "Applying the 1996 JCAHO Nutrition Care Standards in a Long-Term Care Setting." *J Am Diet Assoc* 96(1996): 400–403.
16. Nichols, P. "The Consultant in Health Care Facilities/Extended Care." In: *Dietetics: Practice and Future Trends,* E.A. Winterfeldt, M.L. Bogle, and L.L. Ebro, eds. Gaithersburg, MD: Aspen Publishers, 1998, p. 222.
17. Chidester, J.C., and A.A. Spangler. "Fluid Intake in the Institutionalized Elderly." *J Am Diet Assoc* 97(1997): 23–27.
18. White, J.V., R.J. Ham, D.A. Lipschitz, and J.Y. Dwyer. "Consensus of the Nutrition Screening Initiative: Risk Factors and Indicators of Poor Nutritional Status in Older Americans." *J Am Diet Assoc* 91(1991): 783–787.
19. Gilmore, S.A., G. Robinson, M.E. Posthauer, and J. Raymond. "Clinical Indicators Associated with Unintentional Weight Loss and Pressure Ulcers in Elderly Residents of Nursing Facilities." *J Am Diet Assoc* 95(1995): 984–992.

20. "Quality Management in Hospital-Affiliated Services." In M.R. Schiller, K. Miller-Kovich, and M.A. Miller, eds., *Total Quality Management for Hospital Nutrition Services*. Gaithersburg, MD: Aspen Publishers, 1994.

21. Vogelzang, J.L., and L.L. Roth-Yousey. "Standards of Professional Practice: Measuring the Beliefs and Realities of Consultant Dietitians in Health Care Facilities." *J Am Diet Assoc* 101, no. 4(2001): 473–480.

22. Lechowich, K.A., and T.K. Soto. "Opportunities in Commercial Foodservice: The Industry Perspective." *J Am Diet Assoc* 95(1995): 1163–1166.

23. Davidhizar, R. "Evaluating Creative Management Solutions." *Health Care Sup* 14(1996): 46–49.

24. Rejent-Scholtz, A. "The Growth of Entrepreneurship." In *The Competitive Edge: Advanced Marketing for Dietetic Professionals*. Chicago: The American Dietetic Association, 1995, pp. 8–10.

25. See Note 5.

26. See Note 6.

27. Sneed, J., and J.P. Bukhalter. "Marketing Nutrition in Restaurants: A Survey of Current Practices and Activities." *J Am Diet Assoc* 91(1991): 459–462.

28. Laramee, S.H. "Nutrition Services in Managed Care: New Paradigms for Dietitians." *J Am Diet Assoc* 96(1996): 335–336.

29. Dittoe, A.B. "To Learn the Secret of Success in Business, Listen to Consumer Needs: Marketing the Value of Dietitian's Services." *J Am Diet Assoc* 93(1993): 397–399.

30. Helm, K.K. "Finding Nontraditional Jobs in Dietetics." *J Am Diet Assoc* 91(1991): 419–420.

31. ADA. "Position Paper: Role of the Dietetics Professionals in Health Promotion and Disease Prevention." *J Am Diet Assoc* 102(2002): 1680–1687.

32. Israel, D., and S. Moores. *Beyond Nutrition Counseling: Achieving Positive Outcomes Through Nutrition Therapy*. Chicago, IL: Nutrition Entrepreneurs Dietetic Practice Group, 1996.

33. See Note 5.

34. Rinke, W.J., and S.C. Finn. "Winning Strategies to Excel in Dietetics." *J Am Diet Assoc* 90(1990): 52–58.

35. "Nationwide Nutrition Network Subscription Offer Extended." *ADA Courier* 35, no. 9(1996): 1.

CHAPTER 10

Career Choices in Business, Education, Health, and Wellness

"The ancient Greeks attained a high level of civilization based on good nutrition, regular physical activity, and intellectual development."[1]

Outline

- Introduction
- The Dietitian in Business and Communications
  - New pathways
  - Mentoring and networking
  - Strategic skill building
  - Keeping up to date
- The Dietitian in Health and Wellness Programs
  - Sports, cardiovascular, and wellness dietitians
- The Dietitian in Education and Research
  - Dietitians in education
  - Dietitians in research
  - Career preparation
- Summary

INTRODUCTION

Hospitals and extended care facilities are the work setting for the largest percentage of dietitians and dietetic technicians; however, there are many career choices available to both the entry-level and experienced professional in other settings.

133

Consultation and private practice were discussed in Chapter 9. In this chapter, three areas of practice opportunity are presented: the dietitian in business and communications, in education, and in health and wellness including sports nutrition.

THE DIETITIAN IN BUSINESS
AND COMMUNICATIONS

Following a career path in business and communications has long been considered a nontraditional choice for dietitians. The ADA membership surveys conducted between 1993 and 2002 show that about 30 percent of dietitians work in the for-profit sector, including those in contract food management, managed care organizations, and other for-profit organizations. This for-profit category also represents a wide range of positions including private practice and working with corporations, trade associations, food and pharmaceutical companies, and hotels and restaurants.

In a study of employment trends for dietitians in business and industry, employers (72 percent) as well as prospective employers (62 percent) indicated that the trend toward hiring dietitians is, in fact, increasing. More than 40 percent of employers and their organizations were creating new positions for dietitians. Among the major reasons cited for adding a registered dietitian (RD) to the staff were to increase the company's credibility, to promote the health and nutrition of customers, and to increase the understanding of customer needs.[2] RDs are being hired for positions in sales, marketing, and communications as well.

This trend is likely to continue as consumers become increasingly interested in health promotion and disease prevention. Food Marketing Institute research shows that more than 60 percent of food shoppers are concerned about nutrition, and 45 percent say they are taking more responsibility to ensure that what they eat is nutritious. Although taste remains the number one criterion when choosing food, nutrition is also cited by more than 7 out of 10 shoppers as important in food selection.[3]

New Pathways

There are as many paths to a career in business and communications as there are interested and qualified dietitians to take them. The importance of early exposure to the business world is increasingly recognized through a recommendation that all dietetics students should experience a rotation in a business environment as part of their undergraduate, dietetic internship, or graduate study.[4] Students and supervisors can discover opportunities by contacting exhibitors at professional meetings, local businesses, or by contacting professionals in business and communications. A business rotation may also offer opportunity for exposure to marketing and public relations activities that are essential in business.

How does an individual get a start in business? Several steps are important:[5]

- Make a list of your talents and things you like to do.
- Make a list of all the possible areas into which you could go, including, but not limited to, writing, speaking, publishing, research, marketing, teaching, sales, media, cooking demonstrations, counseling, coaching, managing, catering, and product development.
- Make a list of the population with whom you enjoy working.
- Read newsletters—the ADA journal, dietetic practice group (DPG) newsletters, and other publications—and make a list of dietitians doing things you would enjoy doing.
- Contact those in the areas that seem attractive.
- Talk with other dietitians and find out if they can help make contacts.
- Network, network, network!

Dietitians in business and communications cite several positive things they like about their jobs: challenging work, learning opportunities, opportunity for creativity, fast pace, visibility, and remuneration. At the same time, some indicate there can be stress, long hours, a fast pace, red tape, and a lot of information through which to filter.[6]

To begin investigating a career, the dietitian may refer to the list of business and industry-related group opportunities shown in Table 10–1.

Mentoring and Networking

Dietitians traveling a nontraditional path agree that having a mentor, networking, developing a strategic skill set, and keeping up to date with research and consumer trends are factors necessary to building a successful career. A mentor may be a coworker, an instructor, or another professional. A mentor in the same organization can provide insight into policies, procedures, and the unspoken policies of a company.[7] A mentor can also help an individual see and act on strengths and weaknesses that may affect the job search. The power of mentoring is pointed out in an article in the *Wall Street Journal* stating that 9 out of 10 workers who have received job coaching or mentoring think it is an effective development tool.[8] Some companies have established "inplacement" programs modeled on outplacement techniques to help plan the careers of employees they do not want to lose.

Networking both inside and outside the boundaries of dietetics is a way of finding a mentor, gathering information, and connecting with others.[9] The networking offered through DPGs is invaluable to professionals looking for opportunities for change or advancement in nontraditional areas. Affiliating with other professional associations will provide more ideas and contacts.

Table 10–1   Career Opportunities in Business and Communications

---

Food Industry
  Food and beverage manufacturing and distributing
  Market research companies
  Trade associations
  Hotels and restaurants
  Contract food service companies
  Commodity groups such as the pork, beef, and egg producers
  National associations
    National Dairy Association
    National Livestock and Meat Board
    Food Marketing Institute
    Grocery Manufacturers

Communications
  Freelance writing
  Writing for publications or newsletters
  Public relations and advertising
  Media spokesperson
  Computer training
  Internet education and services

Health Industry Groups
  Worksite wellness programs
  Health clubs and spas
  Pharmaceutical companies
  Nutritional product and dietary supplement companies
  Heart, cancer, and diabetes associations, etc.

Strategic Skill Building

The ability to communicate well, a strong clinical background, and business savvy are three of the strategic skills behind a successful career. In a 1989 ADA study assessing employment trends for dietitians in business and industry, both employers and dietitians ranked communications skills as essential for success.[10] Although dietitians in business and communications may have followed a nontraditional path, it in no way diminishes the importance of their clinical education and experience. For example, if a job requires evaluating research and working with research and development, a good grounding in science is important. An experienced dietitian says: "I prefer to hire dietitians who have some clinical experience. And, they have to be able to understand research before they can report on it."[11] The fundamentals of nutrition therapy are important in learning about people's needs and habits.

Keeping Up to Date

Business and communications are competitive; however, dietitians have skills that are transferable to the business world. Again, successful dietitians in this area of practice say that individuals need to prepare themselves and demonstrate that their acquired skills will fit into the organization. Further, being familiar with the company's products and services and what they are looking for will help the individual's chances of employment. Communication skills are then used to sell oneself.

Advancing into positions with greater responsibility and managerial know-how may require continuing education, often in the business-related areas of study. The growth of online and distance education helps make this possible even for the professional working full-time or in locations away from the educational setting. Dietitians in business frequently continue their education by acquiring an MBA or an advanced degree in management or finance.

Dietitians in business often establish a Web site in order to improve their business image, complement business advertising, attract new clients/customers outside the local area, and start a new business venture.[12] They may also find this a useful tool to learn more about specific businesses and build networks.

THE DIETITIAN IN HEALTH AND WELLNESS PROGRAMS

Wellness, health promotion, corporate fitness, and sports nutrition programs were virtually unheard of 20 years ago. Although both sports and dietetics as professions or areas of interest have existed for centuries, the combination of the two as a career specialty is a relatively recent development. The growth of wellness and fitness programs has been rapid as the relationship between nutritional status and maintenance of health and prevention of disease becomes more evident.[13]

Diet is a known risk factor for the development of the three chronic diseases that are the leading cause of death in adults in the United States: cancer, cardiovascular disease, and stroke.[14] Additional health problems of adults are also closely associated with diet and eating behaviors: obesity, diabetes, high blood pressure, and osteoporosis. Numbers of deaths and medical costs can be significantly altered by changes in diet and lifestyles. Billions of dollars are spent each year on schemes and gimmicks to reduce body weight and prevent cancer, not to mention the money spent in treating adults with these diseases and their complications.

In addition, reports from the National Health and Nutrition Examination Survey III indicate an alarming increase in the prevalence and severity of obesity in young children, older children, and adolescents, as well as adults.[15] These statistics and research point to the need for programs in health promotion, wellness, fitness, and the prevention and treatment of obesity, which greatly expands career options for dietitians.[16] Some dietitians have developed their own programs through practice and research and now market or license the programs to other dietitians and health professionals, both nationally, and internationally. Others continue to work in hospitals, ambulatory care centers, clinics, rehabilitation centers, and athletic clubs or gyms. Those in private practice provide counseling and medical nutrition therapies aimed at preventing and treating obesity.

Even with or perhaps because of the increasing prevalence of obesity, many dietary fads, drugs, and questionable dieting programs have escalated and consume enormous amounts of money each year. This emphasizes the need and opportunities that exist for dietitians and other health professionals in this area.[17]

Sports, Cardiovascular, and Wellness Dietitians

Interest in sports and cardiovascular nutrition among members of the ADA led to the formation in 1981 of the Sports and Cardiovascular Nutritionists (SCAN) DPG of nutrition professionals within the ADA. In 1993, SCAN changed its name to "Sports, Cardiovascular and Wellness Nutritionists" to reflect the importance of wellness and health promotion as a growing area of dietetic practice. In 1994, SCAN welcomed dietetic professionals with an interest in disordered eating into its fold, recognizing the frequent presence of eating disorders among athletes and the critical role that the identification and treatment of disordered eating has in maintaining health and wellness.

The ADA, the Canadian association, and the American College of Sports Nutrition issued a position paper in 2000 concerning nutrition and athletic performance.[18] The importance of optimal nutrition and the roles and responsibilities of health care professionals were discussed in the paper. The educational needs of those aspiring to be sports nutritionists were detailed in an article by Clark in that same ADA journal.[19] Nutrition knowledge, exercise science knowledge, business skills, and a foundation of strong clinical experience are all important, especially because many sports nutritionists are entrepreneurs. A list of the clinical concerns commonly presented to a sports nutritionist is shown in Table 10–2.

Sports Nutrition.   Dietetic professionals with a specialty in sports nutrition can be found in a wide variety of settings from sports medicine clinics to professional football teams, from high school athletics to the Olympics, and from universities to fitness centers.[20] Many incorporate sports nutrition into their more general practice of nutrition counseling or private practice. In the late 1970s, a few entrepreneurial dietitians with interest in sports began offering their services to professional sports teams, often free of charge.[21] Today, several professional teams include dietitians as paid consultants whose expertise serves to enhance the players' performance and

Table 10–2   Clinical Concerns Commonly Presented to a Sports Nutritionist

---

Allergies
Alcohol addiction
Amenorrhea
Anemia
Anorexia
Arteriosclerosis
Binge eating
Body image distortion
Bulimia
Cancer (prevention, recovery from)
Chronic fatigue
Constipation
Diabetes
Diarrhea
Gastric reflux
Gout
Headaches
Hypoglycemia
Hyperlipidemia
Hypertension
Menopause
Obesity/overweight
Osteoporosis
Pregnancy/perinatal nutrition
Stress fractures
Surgery (special nutritional needs pre- and postoperative)

Source: Clark, N. "Identifying the Educational Needs of Aspiring Sports Nutritionists." *J Am Diet Assoc* 100, no. 12(2000): 1522–1524.

---

endurance. A few professional athletes have employed their personal dietitian primarily to help maintain appropriate body weight and ratio of fat to lean body mass.[22]

Some dietitians serve as nutrition trainers for college athletes and teams choosing to specialize in the sport or sports in which they have the greatest personal interest such as swimming, wrestling, baseball, cycling, and others.

The duties and work settings of a sports nutritionist are many and varied and often require irregular work hours such as evenings and weekends. For example, a swim meet may be held all day on a weekend, or a fitness center may offer nutrition classes to its members several evenings a week. A dietitian may occasionally need to travel with a sports team, and this travel may not always be funded by the team.

Many dietetic professionals working in the area of sports nutrition also work as a clinical dietitian for acute care facilities, as outpatient dietitians, or in private practice as nutrition consultants. In addition, some dietitians are employed to supervise the food production and training table in college athletic dormitories. Some professional athletes seek information on eating during off-season to maintain body weight and strength. As part of his or her daily routine, a sports nutritionist may counsel athletes one-on-one regarding their food intake and appropriate nutrients or their use of dietary supplements as ergogenic aids.[23] He or she may also conduct group classes on low-fat eating at a fitness center or work with a high school team to suggest healthful choices for eating on the road. Several sports nutritionists serve as part-time staff at health clubs, available to answer questions members may ask on nutrition or to conduct classes on eating for competition and good health.

An additional career for some dietitians with experience in sports nutrition and fitness has emerged in writing and developing nutrition education materials (newsletters/media shows, and so forth) appropriate for athletes of all ages. Others may enjoy speaking, writing for the media, and consultative arrangements with any number of organizations. Another career option that is growing at the present time has emanated from the proliferation of gymnasiums and physical fitness centers for young children and adolescents. Although started as tumbling and gymnastic opportunities, it is becoming apparent that there is a great need for expertise in nutrition especially combined with the principles of child development. Parents and consumers are welcoming the dietitians' expertise related to obesity, weight maintenance, and disordered eating patterns in young children and adolescents. In some instances, entrepreneurial dietitians are developing centers and mobile units that go to elementary schools or other sites for demonstrations of appropriate physical activity and benefits of good food choices and nutrition.

A knowledge of exercise physiology through course work in exercise science is essential if the sports nutritionist combines nutrition and exercise in working with clients.[24]

Many dietetic professionals seek to enhance their education and expertise by entering graduate programs in exercise physiology, counseling psychology, or business administration. In addition, although few college or university programs in sports nutrition currently exist, many graduate students choose to conduct research for their thesis or dissertation on a topic directly related to sports nutrition. By acquiring a strong foundation in foods and normal and clinical nutrition with study of a related area, the dietetic student can better prepare him- or herself for practice in sports nutrition.

Cardiovascular Nutrition.   With the abundance of research continuing in the area of diet and heart disease, as well as the fact that heart disease remains the number one cause of death for Americans, careers in cardiovascular nutrition offer abundant options.[25] Most acute care facilities whose services include open-heart surgery have cardiac rehabilitation programs in place. These typically include inpatient and outpatient components, both of which offer nutrition counseling and education as part of the program. Cardiac rehabilitation programs offer multidisciplinary teams who deal with all aspects of risk factor reduction, as well as education of the patient and family. Team members may include a medical director, cardiac rehabilitation nurse clinicians, exercise specialist, a physical therapist, a social worker, an occupational therapist, and a dietitian. Education of the patient and families is often conducted in a variety of ways, from individual instruction to group classes. The dietitian may also design and conduct classes on low-fat cooking and other food preparation techniques.

Dietitians who specialize in cardiovascular nutrition may be employed by lipid research clinics. These professionals are responsible for teaching clinic patients how to change their eating habits to lower total fat and saturated fat or to comply with a research feeding protocol. In this setting at a university, they may conduct research on the latest cardiology protocols. Opportunities also exist with pharmaceutical companies as sales representatives or in the public relations departments of large food companies that market products to patients with cardiovascular disease and their families.

Wellness and Health Promotion. The opportunities for dietitians in wellness and health promotion are numerous and diverse. Dietitians who specialize in wellness may have a private practice or consulting business and negotiate contracts with industry, communities, or health clubs. Others are employed by medical centers or corporations to manage their on-site wellness and health promotion programs, which may include conducting classes for employees, developing incentives to foster a greater interest in exercise and nutrition, and increasing productivity by helping to reduce employee illness.[26] Because nutrition is part of wellness, dietitians specializing in wellness and health promotion may also be involved in programs on smoking cessation, meditation and yoga, stress management, exercise, back safety, and employee relations.

Corporations and large institutions initially began providing worksite wellness programs for their employees because research and reports showed that these programs improved the health of employees, increased productivity, and decreased absenteeism and lost work days due to illness.[27] As these programs developed and increased in numbers across the country in businesses of all sizes, data began to accumulate on the economic benefits of worksite wellness programs. With health care costs soaring and major changes occurring in health care and insurance coverages, employers were eager to explore wellness and health promotion programs that would save the corporation money. The common method for defining economic benefits is through the benefit/cost ratio in which the cost is the actual dollar cost of providing the program and benefits are expressed in dollars saved from less absenteeism, reduced disability expenses, and lowered medical costs.

The ability to work as a facilitator and to conduct classes in a group setting are important characteristics of the successful wellness professional. Counseling skills are also necessary, because dealing with high-risk persons may be a regular aspect of the job. In addition, the dietitian must be prepared to analyze and evaluate enormous amounts of information available to employees and clients through media routes: television, newspaper, magazines, and the Internet. This counseling may take place in groups, individually, at health fairs, or even over the telephone.

Wellness and fitness programs are emerging for the aging and retired population as well as the younger employed groups. Research is indicating that even though aging is inevitable, biologic aging can be delayed through appropriate nutrition and exercise.[28] As the number of senior citizens increases, this will provide another career opportunity for dietitians specializing in health promotion. Fitness programs including nutrition, exercise, and lifestyle changes are developing that improve the quality of life and encourage wellness in this age group.

Several national organizations provide excellent and accurate information for the dietitian seeking up-to-date knowledge on wellness and health promotion programs and concepts. In addition, all have information on the Internet. The major organizations are listed with Internet addresses:

- The American Dietetic Association (www.eatright.org)
- International Food Information Council (ificinfo.health.org)
- National Institutes of Health (NIH) National Cancer Institute 5 a Day Program (www.dcpc.nci.nih.gov/5aday)
- President's Council on Physical Fitness and Sports (www.os.dhhs.gov)
- Centers for Disease Control and Prevention (CDC) National Center for Chronic Disease Prevention and Health Promotion (www.cdc.gov/nccdphp)
- American College of Sports Medicine (www.csm.org)
- American Alliance on Health, Physical Education, Recreation, and Dance (www.ashperd.org)

The Internet also offers the opportunity and challenge for the individual dietitian to develop Web sites and disseminate nutrition and fitness messages by this means.

Disordered Eating. Dietitians who specialize in disordered eating work in a variety of settings, including residential treatment centers, hospitals (both medical and psychiatric), outpatient clinics, managed care organizations, university health centers, and private practice. The specialty of disordered or problematic eating encompasses several areas in which nutritional, physical, and psychological issues are intertwined with eating behavior, such as obesity, chronic dieting, anorexia nervosa, bulimia nervosa, compulsive eating, and binge eating disorders.[29] Complications of these disorders are potentially life threatening. Many have their origin or manifestation in childhood or adolescence. Although most of these disorders affect adolescent females, there have been a few reports of similar behavior in males. Effective treatment of disordered eating required knowledge and skills in counseling, cognitive behavioral therapy, family systems theory, addiction, and psychopharmacology.[30]

Because of the biopsychosocial nature of disordered eating, the role of the dietitian on the treatment team is vital. The dietitian educates the client about food, physical activity, and body size and shape and guides him or her in developing a sound eating style and physical activity pattern. Clients may share their thoughts and feelings about food, weight, and physical activity with the dietitian. They may also share life situations and events that are stressful for them, such as job change, marital problems, school problems, relationships, and burnout. The dietitian helps clients identify how stress affects their eating style and how they feel about food, their body size, and shape, and physical activity.[31] Ongoing communication with the treatment team therapist, psychiatrist, and physician is essential so that the dietitian can discern which issues are nutrition related and which are psychological or medical. It takes years of experience for the dietitian to most effectively complement his or her skills and expertise with other members of the team.

Dietitians working in programs to treat disordered eating benefit from regular supervision from a mental health professional who specializes in problematic eating. This provides a forum for discussion of specific cases, as well as helping to clarify which issues are appropriately addressed in nutrition therapy versus psychotherapy. Furthermore, many dietitians are seeking continuing education in areas such as women's issues, cognitive behavioral therapy, family counseling, psychotherapeutic counseling skills, and psychopharmacology. The intention is to sharpen counseling skills and enhance the understanding of sociologic and psychological aspects of disordered eating, while consistently staying within the scope of practice of the dietetic professional.

THE DIETITIAN IN EDUCATION AND RESEARCH

Almost every dietitian serves as an educator some of the time. For example, the dietitian in food services conducts in-service programs for employees, and public health nutritionists give classes for home care nurses. Clinical dietitians participate in medical nutrition education, and they often conduct group classes for patients with diabetes or coronary heart disease. Consultant dietitians may give food demonstrations for chefs. Dietitians working with Women, Infants, and Children food programs may teach Head Start children how to prevent or reduce the incidence of obesity and adult-onset diabetes.[32] In industry, dietitians are called on to teach sales representatives about specialty nutrition products. Many dietitians are preceptors for dietetics students. Dietitians in every area of practice give classes during national nutrition month; yet, these dietetics practitioners are unlikely to classify themselves as "educators."

Many dietitians conduct research as a part of their work. This is especially true for dietitians who specialize in nutrition support, pediatrics, renal dietetics, oncology, acquired immunodeficiency syndrome (AIDS), diabetes, or other clinical subspecialties. Such dietitians often critique research articles or collect research data. They are encouraged to do outcome research studies to demonstrate the effectiveness of medical nutrition therapy. They may collaborate with physicians who are conducting nutrition-related studies. However, these dietitians are unlikely to call themselves "researchers."

This discussion focuses on full-time career opportunities in education and research and offers a bird's eye view of teaching and research positions in schools, colleges and universities, medical centers, government agencies, and industry.

Dietitians in Education

Elementary and Secondary Schools.   Most school-based nutrition education is incorporated into health and science classes in primary, middle, and high schools. A dietitian who teaches at these levels needs to meet state teacher training and certification requirements. Generally, those who teach grades K-12 have responsibilities that extend well beyond food, nutrition, and health.

Some state departments of education have nutrition education and training sections that often employ registered dietitians who have advanced degrees in education. Such positions include creating curricula to integrate nutrition with other subjects, developing teaching materials, identifying instructional resources, and training teachers to deliver nutrition education.[33]

Job opportunities for dietitians in child nutrition programs affect dietitians from the lunchroom to the classroom. School-based health centers—rapidly growing models for the delivery of comprehensive, primary health care to elementary, middle, and senior high school students—afford another opportunity for dietitians interested in working with children and adolescents.[34]

Colleges and Universities.   There are teaching opportunities for dietitians in culinary institutes, technical schools, and 2- and 4-year colleges. Such positions are often associated with programs for chefs, food service supervisors, dietetic technicians, dietary managers, entry-level dietitians, and hospitality managers. The emphasis is on teaching in the classroom, laboratory, or practice setting. Course responsibilities may include food preparation and food science, basic and applied nutrition, meal management, cultural food practices, food service management and equipment, nutrition assessment and therapy, nutrition counseling and education, and community nutrition.

University faculty roles are quite varied. In addition to their teaching responsibilities, university faculty are required to conduct research and provide service within the institution, community, or profession. They spend time advising students on academic choices and research, serving on committees, consulting with community groups, sharing their expertise with the media and the public, and providing leadership for nutrition-related initiatives.

Higher education can include teaching other groups of students. For example, some institutions offer nutrition courses for nondietitian majors to fulfill requirements for general education, teacher certification, or health and physical education. Programs in the allied health professions may include nutrition courses. Dietitians can teach courses in nutritional anthropology or epidemiology, often included as part of masters in public health programs.

Medical and Dental Education.   Some graduate-trained dietitians are engaged in medical and dental education. Such a role requires assertiveness and creativity to convince administrators of the unique role that dietitians can play in this regard. Besides an in-depth knowledge of nutrition science and medical nutrition therapy, medical and dental nutrition educators must possess leadership, self-direction, strong communication skills, conceptual thinking skills, time management, and flexibility.[35]

Nutrition education can occur at any level of a medical or dental curriculum. It may consist of nutrition science with clinical applications during the first 2 years. As students enter the clinical part of their program, sample meals featuring special diets are effective.[36] Nutrition rounds and seminars can be incorporated when students are in residencies. Practicing dietitians can be involved in problem-based learning as an effective way to make nutrition relevant for future medical practice.[37]

Nursing and Allied Health Nutrition Education.   Nutrition services are often provided by nondietitians, depending on the practice setting and contributions of various health professionals. For example, nurses regularly monitor food intake, evaluate laboratory values indicative of nutritional status, and give patients nutritional advice.[38] Dental hygienists and health educators often screen for health or nutritional problems and provide education and intervention. All health professionals should understand the role nutrition plays in wellness and disease prevention, and they need training on appropriate interventions. It is generally agreed that nutrition education for nurses and other health professionals should be increased.[39]

The ADA supports nutrition education for the health professions and advocates including the inclusion of nutrition in didactic, clinical, and continuing education programs.[40] Dietitians are prepared to provide leadership for such programs and to direct nutrition education efforts in schools of nursing, pharmacy, allied health, and social work. However, there is a shortage of qualified faculty in this area.

Industry-Based Education.   Companies that manufacture medical nutrition products often employ dietitians to provide technical and clinical information to the sales force and to other personnel, clinicians, retail pharmacists, and educators of health care professionals. Dietitians may educate via telephone, written correspondence, and electronic mail. They may organize educational conferences and disseminate proceedings. They may participate in developing video, audio, and slide programs; technical monographs; newsletters; brochures; and professional and patient education publications on topics of medical nutrition therapy.[41]

Personal characteristics and skills necessary for success in industry-based education include "technical and professional proficiency, ability to critically and objectively analyze issues, attention to detail, high work standards, skill at written and oral communication, adaptability, and ability to tolerate stress.[42] Clearly, such positions require a proficiency in nutritional sciences, practitioner experience, conceptual and analytic skills, altruistic values, and service ethic.

Worksite Nutrition Education.   As increased attention is given to the role of nutrition in health and disease prevention, there will be more opportunities for dietitians in worksite wellness programs. These worksites may include manufacturing plants, insurance companies, or service organizations. Some of these positions will focus entirely on nutrition education and may include screening for nutritional risk, developing programs, giving classes and demonstrations, creating exhibits and displays, and evaluating the effectiveness of nutrition education initiatives. Dietitians in these positions may provide valuable experience for dietetic interns or other students.[43]

Worksite education opportunities can also include coordinators of training in large dietetics departments or at the regional level of contract food and nutrition service companies. Dietitians in such roles may oversee a dietetic internship, coordinate in-service training for food service and other personnel, and direct training for students from affiliating programs. Individuals with the appropriate background may be promoted to director of training and development at the institutional or corporate level.

Dietitians in Research

Much of the research in nutrition and dietetics is conducted by students and faculty members in colleges and universities. Some of these researchers are registered dietitians; others are food or nutrition scientists. Most faculty members are in research as well as teaching as part of their faculty responsibilities. They may conduct laboratory research such as metabolic studies in human nutrient requirements or in food science to determine the utilization of specific food components. Other studies may be conducted in controlled working environments as, for example, in food service management productivity studies. Other types of research may deal with applied studies in nutrition education and data collection through surveys. Further career opportunities for dietitians in research are described in Chapter 13.

Career Preparation

One or more years practicing in a hospital, nursing home, clinic, or community setting is the first step toward success as a dietitian in education and/or research. Those with first-hand experience in the field gain a valuable understanding of the practice milieu, and they can draw from these backgrounds for illustrations and examples.

Interest in research can develop early. Fundamental skill development often begins with an undergraduate research course, completion of an honors research study, or summer work in a research laboratory. Nearly all dietitians in education and research have attained at least a masters degree, and many have earned a doctorate. In addition, these individuals tend to be creative, intellectually curious, and self-directed achievers. They love libraries and they enjoy working at a scholarly level. Because much of their work involves communication and motivating others, they must have good interpersonal skills and a sense of humor.

Education and Research Practice Groups   Dietitians in education and research have numerous opportunities to unite with colleagues having similar interests (see Table 10–3). As noted earlier, the ADA practice groups promote networking, mentoring, information exchange, professional enhancement, and leadership opportunities in organized areas of practice. Generally, practice groups offer their members continuing education programs, quarterly newsletters, forums for exploring practice issues, and innovative products and services.

Table 10–3   Purpose of ADA Practice Groups for Dietitians in Research and Education

Nutrition Research Practice Group
   Promotes visibility of nutrition research and communication between researchers and practitioners.
Dietetic Educators of Practitioners
   Unites members of ADA who are interested in or engaged in educating dietitians and dietetic technicians; represents the concerns of dietetic educators to the ADA, the government, institutions of higher learning, and the public.
Nutrition Educators of Health Professionals
   Advocates improvement in the quality of nutrition education of medical, dental, nursing, and allied health students; provides a forum for communication and information exchange between members, especially new educators; offers expertise in the development of nutrition curricula for undergraduate and graduate education.
Nutrition Education for the Public
   Champions improved well-being of the public by providing leadership in nutrition education planning, implementation, and evaluation; provides members with resources and opportunities to enhance both personal skills and nutrition expertise.

Source: Adapted with permission from *Dietetics Practice Group Information.* American Dietetic Association.

Both education and research are essential for advancement of the dietetics profession. To prepare for these careers, students are encouraged to become associate members of ADA, join relevant ADA practice groups, seek career advice or mentoring from dietitians in education and research, enroll in pertinent elective courses, and begin planning for graduate study.

Opportunities in education and research are available in many areas of practice. Experience and advanced study are usual requirements for practice.

SUMMARY

Dietitians with expertise in worksite wellness, sports and cardiovascular nutrition, and disordered eating are increasingly in demand in nontraditional settings. They must be creative and adept in the promotion of healthy eating behaviors. In addition, the nutrition education must be presented in a manner that is sensitive to the client's age, cultural background, and level of education. He or she must also be able to translate scientific information into "user-friendly" terms.

DEFINITIONS

Academic Health Centers. Hospitals, medical centers, or clinics affiliated with a
   medical school or medical residency program.
Anorexia Nervosa. The eating disorder in which preoccupation with dieting and
   thinness leads to excessive weight loss.
Bulimia Nervosa. The eating disorder involving frequent episodes of binge eating
   and nearly always followed by purging.
Cardiovascular Nutrition. Application of medical nutrition therapy for those with
   heart and blood vessel conditions or to prevent the diseases.
Disordered Eating. Abnormal eating patterns.
Health Promotion. Education and preventive measures directed toward basically
   healthy populations to foster wellness.
Networking. Activities directed toward making connections with others through
   varied contacts.
Nontraditional Job. Job or position outside the usual or most common areas of
   practice.
Sports Nutrition. The area of nutrition specific to the needs of those who participate in sports activities.
Value System. Set of principles guiding actions that adhere to professional and
   ethical practice.
Wellness. State of optimal health and the absence of disease.

REFERENCES

1. Simopoulos, A. "Declaration of Olympia on Nutrition and Fitness." *Nutr Today* 3(1996): 250–252.

2. Kirk, D., C.W. Shanklin, and M.A. Gorman. "Attributes and Qualifications That Employers Seek When Hiring Dietitians in Business and Industry." *J Am Diet Assoc* 89(1989): 494–498.

3. Kapica, C., and J.O.S. Maillet. "A Business Rotation for Dietitians—An Imperative in the New Millennium." *J Am Diet Assoc* 1029(2002): 1220.

4. *Trends in the United States: Consumer Attitudes and the Supermarket, 1995.* Washington, DC: Food Marketing Institute, 1995.

5. Indorato, D.A. "Innovative Services by and for Dietitians." *Today's Diet* 3, no. 4(2001): 16–19.

6. Informal survey of dietitians working in business and communications, February 1996.

7. Finn, S.C. "The Dietitian in Business and Communications." In *Dietetics Practice and Future Trends,* E.A. Winterfeldt, M. Bogle, and L.L. Ebro, eds. Gaithersburg, MD: Aspen Publishers, 1998, p. 249.

8. Business Briefing. "'Inplacement' Programs." *Wall St J.* December 14, 1995, p. A1.

9. See Note 5.

10. See Note 2.

11. Finn, S.C. "The Dietitian in Business and Communications." In *Dietetics Practice and Future Trends,* E.A. Winterfeldt, M. Bogle, and L.L. Ebro, eds. Gaithersburg, MD: Aspen Publishers, 1998, p. 251.

12. Pangan, T., and C. Bedner. "Dietitian Business Websites: A Survey of Their Profitability and How You Can Make Yours Profitable." *J Am Diet Assoc* 101, no. 4(2001): 399–402.

13. Public Health Service. "The Surgeon General's Report on Nutrition and Health, 1988." Washington, DC: U.S. Department of Health and Human Services, 1988. DHHS Pub. PH S88-50210.

14. Troiano, R.P., K.M. Flegal, R.J. Kuczmarski, and S.M. Campbell. "Overweight Prevalence and Trends for Children and Adolescents: The National Health and Nutrition Examination Surveys, 1963–1991." *Arch Pediatr Adolesc Medicine* 149(1995): 1085–1091.

15. Please supply reference.

15. Burns, R.D., M.R. Schiller, M.A. Merrick, and K.N. Wolf. "Intercollegiate Student Athlete Use of Nutritional Supplements and the Role of Athletic Trainers and Dietitians in Nutrition Counseling." *J Am Diet Assoc* 104, no. 2(2004): 246–249.

16. Heaton, A.W., and A.S. Leng. "Information Sources of U.S. Adults Trying to Lose Weight." *J Nutr Educ* 27(1995): 182–190.

17. ADA. "Position of the American Dietetic Association: Dietitians of Canada and the American College of Sports Medicine: Nutrition and Athletic Performance." *J Am Diet Assoc* 100, no. 12(2000): 1543–1556.

18. Clark, N. "Identifying the Educational Needs of Aspiring Sports Nutritionist." *J Am Diet Assoc* 100, no. 12(2000): 1522–1524.

19. Shattuck, D. "Sports Nutritionists Feel the Competitive Edge." *J Am Diet Assoc* 101, no. 5(2001): 517–518.

20. Grandjean, A.C. "Diet of Elite Athletes: Has the Discipline of Sports Nutrition Made an Impact?" *J Nutr* 127(1997): 874S–877S.

21. Tipton, C.M. "Sports Medicine: A Century of Progress." *J Nutr* 127(1997): 878S–885S.

22. Applegate, E.A., and L.E. Grivetti. "Search for the Competitive Edge: A History of Dietary Fads and Supplements." *J Nutr* 127(1997): 869S–873S.

23. See Note 19.

24. Messer, J., and W. Stone. "Worksite Fitness and Health Promotion Benefit/Cost Analysis: A Tutorial, Review of Literature, and Assessment of the State of the Art. *Worksite Health* 2(1995): 34–43.

25. Kaman, R.L., ed. *Worksite Health Promotion Economics: Consensus and Analysis.* Champaign, IL: Human Kinetic Publishers, 1995.

26. Ibid.

27. Evans, W.J., and D. Cyr-Campbell. "Nutrition, Exercise, and Healthy Aging." *J Am Diet Assoc* 97(1997): 632–638.

28. Seymour, M., S.L. Hoerr, and Y.L. Huang. "Inappropriate Dieting Behavior and Related Lifestyle Factors in Young Adults: Are College Students Different?" *J Nutr Educ* 29(1997): 21–26.

29. Ammerman, S.D., G.H. Shih, and J. Ammerman. "Unique Considerations for Treating Eating Disorders in Adolescents and Preventive Intervention." *Topics in Clin Nutr* 12(1996): 79–85.

30. Fisher, M., N.H. Golden, and D.K. Katzman. "Eating Disorders in Adolescents: A Background Paper." *J Adolesc Health* 16(1995): 420–437.

31. Rubin, K.W. "Creative Nutrition Education for Headstart Children of the Seminole Tribe of Florida." *Topics in Clin Nutr* 9(1994): 73–78.

32. Shannon, B., R. Mullis, V. Bernardo, and B. Ervin. "The Status of School-Based Nutrition at the State Agency Level." *J School Health* 62(1992): 88–92.

33. Juszczak, L., M. Fisher, J.C. Lear, and S.B. Friedman. "Back to School: Training Opportunities in School-Based Health Centers." *J Dev Behav Pediatr* 16(1995): L101–104.

34. Kolasa, K.M., and A.B. Lasswell. "Dietitians as Medical Educators." *Topics in Clin Nutr* 10(1995): 20–28.

35. Tillman, H.H., M. Woods, and S.L. Gorbach. "Enhancing the Level of Nutrition Education at Tufts University's Medical and Dental Schools." *J Cancer Educ* 7(1992): 215–219.

36. Reiter, S.A., D.N. Rasmann-Nuhlicek, K. Biernat, and S.L. Lawrence. "Registered Dietitians as Problem-Based Learning Facilitators in a Nutrition Curriculum for Freshman Medical Students." *J Am Diet Assoc* 94(1994): 652-654.

37. Weigley, E.S. "Nutrition in Nursing Education and Beginning Practice." *J Am Diet Assoc* 94(1994): 654–656.

38. Englert, D.A.M., K.S. Crocker, and N.A. Stotts. "Nutrition Education in Schools of Nursing in the United States. Part I: The Evolution of Nutrition Education in Schools of Nursing." *JPEN* 10(1986): 522–527.

39. ADA. "Position of the American Dietetic Association: Nutrition Education of Health Professionals." *J Am Diet Assoc* 91(1991): 611–613.

40. Campbell, S.M. "Looking for Wonder Woman: A Role for Registered Dietitians in Industry-Based Education." *Topics in Clin Nutr* 10(1995): 14–19.

41. Sandoval, W.M., and H.D. Mueller. "Nutrition Education at the Worksite: A Team Approach." *J Am Diet Assoc* 89(1989): 543–544.

42. Ibid.

PART IV

Roles Essential for Dietitians

CHAPTER 11

The Dietitian as Manager and Leader

"Skills such as team building, delegation, communication, negotiation, and self-management are fundamental to high performance. Fortunately, these can be learned and enhanced through continuing education and training."[1]

Outline

- Introduction
- Management and Leadership
- Leadership
  — Attaining leadership skills
- Management Functions
- Skills and Abilities of Managers
  — Human relations skills
  — Technical skills
  — Conceptual skills
- Further Management Roles
- Summary

INTRODUCTION

Management is often thought of as those activities that have to do with "being in charge" or being "the boss" of a department or an institution with many responsibilities; therefore, the entry-level dietitian does not need to be concerned with knowing how to manage. In reality, all dietitians, regardless of their job title or job responsibilities, perform many managerial functions and need to develop managerial skills. The clinical dietitian, the food service management dietitian, the nutritionist in community nutrition programs, the educator, the private practitioner, and the dietitian in business all perform management functions. Among these functions are management of resources, assessing performance, training others, setting goals, communicating, and practicing quality control.

In this chapter, we discuss management and leadership functions and skills and illustrate how each relates to professional practice in dietetics.

MANAGEMENT AND LEADERSHIP

Management and leadership have many overlapping characteristics, but they are not the same.[2] The manager must make things happen, must function as an operator of a department or unit, and will use many leadership activities to do so. Some skills, however, are unique to the leader. In Table 11–1, several activities are illustrated that balance management and leadership.

LEADERSHIP

Drucker points out that leadership is a means to an end—not just a quality to be desired. He considers the three most important characteristics for successful leadership are:[3]

1. The foundation of effective leadership is thinking through the organization's mission, defining it, and establishing it clearly and visibly. The leader sets

Table 11–1   Balancing Management and Leadership

The Focus on Management	The Vision of Leadership
Do things right	Do the right things
Direct operations	Monitor guest expectations
Enforce policies and rules	Communicate vision and values
Design procedures and tasks	Manage systems and processes
Control results	Support people
Foster stability	Engage in continuous improvement

Source: Woods, R.H., and J.Z. King. *Quality Leadership and Management in the Hospitality Industry.* East Lansing, MI: Educational Institute of the American Hotel and Motel Association, 1996, p. 20.

the goals, the priorities, and maintains the standards. He or she makes compromises as necessary.

2. The leader sees leadership as a responsibility and not a rank or privilege. Effective leaders are rarely permissive, but when things go wrong, they do not blame others. They encourage and help develop strong associates and subordinates..

3. The effective leader must earn trust in order to have followers. To trust a leader, it is not necessary to like or to agree; rather trust is the conviction that the leader means what he or she says and has integrity.

Crucial activities that are characteristic of the successful leader in terms of managerial roles are shown in Table 11–2.

Several theories of leadership and leadership styles are discussed in the book *Leadership in Dietetics.*[4] All dietitians will benefit from the examples of leadership in action outlined in this book.

Attaining Leadership Skills

The question as to whether people are born leaders or whether they develop the leadership skills to become leaders has proponents for both views. In support of the supposition that leadership skills can be acquired, several actions that are characteristic of the effective leader include the following:[5]

- Be creative by encouraging innovative staff performance, involving subordinates in decision making, and rewarding them for contributions.
- Form teams that will foster employee satisfaction, personal mastery, empowerment, and effective problem solving.
- Take risks by showing that it is acceptable to try nontraditional methods, thereby fostering ingenuity and resourcefulness.
- Expect failure and state this to subordinates so they know that creativity cannot be hampered by fear of failure.
- Encourage continuous learning so that higher levels of competence and responsibility can be achieved.
- Communicate effectively so that trust within teams and high performance are promoted.
- Symbolize the unit's activities by demonstrating knowledge of how "things work."
- Benchmark by comparing performance with that of other operators and finding better methods and systems through sharing information with colleagues. This will provide further ideas for planning.
- Walk around, be visible, and be involved with the daily activities of the unit.

Table 11–2   Thirty Crucial Activities for the Successful Leader

Role Set	Mintzberg's (1980) 10 Managerial Roles	30 Crucial Activities
Motivating others	Figurehead Liaison Leader	1. Recruiting professionals 2. Making decisions regarding professionals and managerial salaries 3. Devising work procedures for professionals 4. Devising work procedures for nonprofessionals 5. Promoting and rewarding professionals and managers 6. Conducting employee and management development and training 7. Disciplining professional and managerial employees 8. Motivating and directing immediate subordinates 9. Dealing with personal and interpersonal problems
Scanning the environment	Monitor Disseminator	10. Market research 11. Product research 12. Long-range planning 13. Criteria systems development to control quality 14. Decisions regarding financial and management information systems
Negotiating the political terrain	Spokesperson Negotiator Disturbance handler	15. Conducting public relations 16. Lobbying 17. Conducting labor negotiations 18. Establishing agreements with other institutions 19. Negotiating with powerful external organizations 20. Creating and changing professional job unity 21. Making decisions regarding changes in decision-making and authority structure 22. Influencing decisions of administration or the board 23. Influencing decisions made by the medical staff 24. Arbitrating between internal units and/or other departments
Generating and allocating resources	Entrepreneur Resource allocator	25. Decisions regarding buying procedure 26. Decisions regarding working capital expenses

Table 11–2 continued

Role Set	Mintzberg's (1980) 10 Managerial Roles	30 Crucial Activities
		27. Decisions regarding maintaining building and equipment
		28. Decisions regarding charges and prices for services
		29. Decisions regarding new construction
		30. Decisions regarding general operation

Source: Jackson, R. *Nutrition and Food Services for Integrated Health Care: A Handbook for Leaders.* Gaithersburg, MD: Aspen Publishers, 1997, p. 74.

MANAGEMENT FUNCTIONS

Management is often defined in terms of the traditional functions that various management experts have described and written about over the years. Although the number of functions may vary according to the way in which they are presented, the following six functions are universally accepted:[6]

1. *Planning* is the activity of setting goals and objectives. The extent of the planning, from setting broad, long-range goals for a large organization to planning shorter-term goals, will usually be determined by where persons are in the organizational hierarchy.
2. *Organizing* is the reflection of how the organization accomplishes its goals and objectives. The tasks to be performed, the assignment of the tasks, allocation of resources, and the flow of authority and communication are established.
3. *Coordinating* involves activities that lead to the efficient use of resources to attain the noted goals and objectives.
4. *Staffing* means determining human resource needs, then recruiting, selecting, hiring, and training the necessary staff.
5. *Directing* (or *leading*) refers to those activities that accomplish the organization goals, communicate those goals, and create an atmosphere that encourages commitment and desired performance.
6. *Controlling* occurs when performance is assessed against standards that have been translated from the goals and objectives and applying corrective measures as needed.

SKILLS AND ABILITIES OF MANAGERS

The particular skills needed by managers to effectively function are often grouped into three types: *human relations, technical, and conceptual* (see Figures 11–1A and B).

As indicated in these figures, earlier traditional views of management held that top managers primarily needed human relations and conceptual skills, while the more contemporary view is that technical skills are increasingly important for the top manager, especially in small organizations and in those with flattened and decentralized organization patterns. Middle managers require an almost equal distribution of skills among the three types, while the supervisor is viewed as needing slightly more conceptual skills than earlier. In the contemporary view, workers in the organization also need all skills, but the emphasis is on the technical. The use of particular skills will vary from day to day with changes in the work environment such as the need to hire and train new employees or to engage in long-range strategic planning.

Human Relations Skills

Personal Relationships.   Interpersonal skills are always rated highly when management skills are described or studied. The ability to work with others toward common goals is the number one factor denoting success among health care multidepartmental managers.[7] Numerous books and articles have been published about establishing and maintaining interpersonal relationships. Every dietitian will benefit from one or more in his or her library. The *Harvard Business Review* is also an excellent source for readings in this area.

"Generational diversity" or the involvement of several distinct generations in the workplace presents another aspect of achieving successful working relationships.[8] Different generations of workers are assumed to have different loyalties and expectations resulting in the need for open-mindedness, effective communications, and respect for others.

Communications.   Communication at both an organizational and a personal level is an essential part of every manager's job. Two excellent references concerning communications include *Communicating as Professionals*[9] and *Communication and Education Skills: The Dietitian's Guide.*[10]

Verbal and nonverbal skills as well as listening skills are vital to know and practice. Because communicating online has become an important means of communication in all areas of practice, dietitians need to be aware of ways to create, access, share, and use online information fully and effectively.[11]

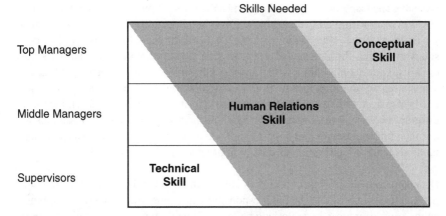

Figure 11–1A   Traditional Cross Section of Management Skills. *Source:* Woods, R.H., and J.Z. King. *Quality Leaderships and Management in the Hospitality Industry.* East Lansing, MI: Educational Institute of the American Hotel and Motel Association, 1996, p. 16.

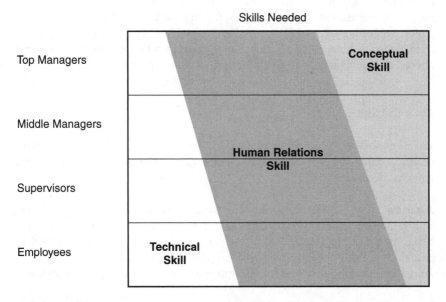

Figure 11–1B   Contemporary Cross Section of Management Skills. *Source:* Woods, R.H., and J.Z. King. *Quality Leaderships and Management in the Hospitality Industry.* East Lansing, MI: Educational Institute of the American Hotel and Motel Association, 1996, p. 16.

Coaching and Mentoring.   Most dietitians will at some time in their career be in the position of assisting and supporting a coworker or employee as they learn a new job or develop new skills and will become a coach or a mentor. A *mentor* is a person who teaches through verbal instructing, demonstration of particular activities or skills, and role modeling, while the *coach* is one who inspires and motivates.[12] The successful dietitian in a work unit may function in either of these capacities in order to accomplish needed tasks. Staff perform at different levels and learn in different ways. It is the enterprising coach or mentor who is able to adapt actions to motivate, encourage, and support staff, thereby creating a productive and harmonious team. Mentoring is discussed in greater detail in Chapter 12.

Managing Conflict.   Conflict occurs in any organization and may result from competition for resources, overlapping responsibilities, status struggles, poor communications, or differences in values and beliefs.[13] The dietitian who recognizes causes of conflict and assists in taking steps to overcome the differences will be looked to as a manager/leader.

Networking.   Networking within an organization leads to interconnectedness. People form networks for sharing social and business information and to increase professional competence. The manager/leader will seek opportunities to network and will further encourage others in the work unit to network. Networking with other professionals through the dietetic practice groups of the American Dietetic Association (ADA) and other groups can lead to personal growth, a greater understanding of practice requirements, and enhanced performance in every area of practice.

Technical Skills

Technical skills are those that require a specialized knowledge of techniques, methods, procedures, and processes that accomplish the work of an organization. Several types are discussed:

Job Skills.   The manager/leader has knowledge of what is required to perform in an organization but may not actually perform the work except on an "as-needed" basis. Instead, the knowledge allows the manager to supervise those with the specific skills to fulfill the job requirements. The need to have job "know-how" is essential for assessing performance, meeting goals, and ensuring quality outputs.

Resource Management.   Financial management including cost controls comes to mind first when the management of resources is described as a management function. Resources, however, can also mean job-related supplies and equipment, staff assistance, and even time and energy. Every dietitian and dietetic technician carries certain responsibilities for managing these types of resources and may also be involved in budgeting and long-range planning.

Activities related to maintaining cost-effectiveness and cost controls are familiar to all professionals. An ADA position paper[14] affirms the role of the clinical dietetics professional in cost containment in order to show the economic benefits of medical nutrition therapy.

The importance of teaching financial management in dietetics programs is emphasized by dietetics program directors. In one survey, educators agreed or strongly agreed with the statement: "Entry-level registered dietitians need to be trained in financial management concepts as well as clinical concepts in order to be competent practitioners."[15]

Benchmarking is a process used to measure the efficiency of work, the products produced, and the services for comparison and improvement.[16] It is used effectively in both health care and in food services. Performance measures including financial, customer services, human resources, and operational are usually evaluated in the benchmarking process. Measurements are used that provide information that may then be compared and used for improvement.

Training and Staff Development. The responsibility for hiring and training a workforce is primarily that of upper-level management. However, all professionals will at times help train and develop new employees or other professionals. The team concept often followed in health care institutions as well as in food service and hospitality requires that all members of a team function fully and efficiently. Further, team members must know their job-related roles as well as their expected role as a team member. Efficiency evolves from knowledge and practice and must be encouraged and assisted by those already experienced within an organization.

Technology Know-How. The importance of communication has been discussed as a human relations skill. Knowing how to access and use all available technological means of communication is a must for all professionals in the modern workplace. Online information is rapidly becoming the means by which most professionals stay current. Conferences, workshops, meetings, and classes are increasingly offered by teleconference or online or by similar means using newer technology.

Not only is communications technology of increasing importance, but technology related to better and faster job performance benefits both individuals and an organization. To the extent that professionals become experts in the technology needed for their jobs, they will also become mentors and coaches for others.

Team Building. A team functions in ways that support individual efforts and leads to greater productivity. Teams vary in number, may be formal or informally organized, and may be formed in a variety of ways. For instance, a team may be formed within a department or from several departments or disciplines to accomplish more than can be accomplished by individuals. Teams may also be temporary or permanent.

The value of teams lies in sharing knowledge and working toward common goals using the experience and expertise of several in decision making and problem solving. The manager/leader encourages teams and helps make them effective by arranging for persons to participate and providing for training of team members as needed. Teams function best when they are empowered with authority or legal power to reach a level of self-management.[17]

Work groups are often formed of persons working together for an organizational purpose.[18] As with teams, they may be formally constituted or may function in a more informal way such as a gathering of people to solve daily problems. The group leader has several tasks, that include understanding the internal workings of the group, planning ahead and being proactive, and managing interpersonal relations for cohesiveness of the group.

Quality Management.   *Quality* is a term defined as meeting standards and expectations; sometimes in terms of high quality or above a norm or average. Quality health care has been defined as:

> "the degree to which health services for individuals and populations increase the likelihood of desired health outcomes and are consistent with current professional knowledge. Dimensions of quality include the following: patient perspective issues, safety of the care environment, and accessibility, appropriateness, continuity, efficiency, efficacy, and timeliness of the care."[19]

Every institution, department, business, or professional association strives to "produce" quality goods, services, or people. Rather than relying on subjective methods to detect quality, most organizations establish performance measures by which they assess and ensure continuous quality.

In every area of dietetics, performance standards are in effect and are described in other sections of this book. Food production managers use performance measures to ensure the quality of the food service. Patient satisfaction surveys are used in continuous assessment of the service received. Clinical outcomes can be measured for quality through specific agreed-on indicators. The community nutritionist measures quality of services by satisfactory outcomes of persons receiving instruction and care. The educator measures outcomes and the quality of the education by how their students perform.

Even though "quality" is a somewhat elusive descriptor, it is a part of every dietitian's job responsibility and is a managerial function.

Conceptual Skills

The manager/leader performs a certain number of activities based on thinking about the bigger picture beyond the technical aspects of his or her position. The ability to visualize long range, to plan and set goals, to provide direction in an organization, and to model professional behavior constitutes conceptual ability or skill.

Strategic Planning and Goal Setting. In general, strategic planning occurs at the upper levels of management because it requires data gathering and data analysis, development of strategies and goals and objectives, and implementation of action plans. However, professionals at all levels in an organization participate in data gathering and in setting short- and long-term goals. They are a part of the planning process that occurs in an organization that sets direction and a plan of action.

Some plans are general such as the determination of value, mission, and vision statements.[20] Others are more detailed and may be developed at supervisory levels. If operational plans are short range, they are usually expected to occur within a year: long-term plans extend beyond a year and up to 10 years. The food and nutrition professional often contributes to both types of planning by conducting feasibility studies, cost-effectiveness studies, and quality-control measures.

One description of planning for *patient-focused* care, using health care teams, gives examples of a model for patient care through a multiskilled approach.[21] The clinical supervisor and clinical staff are closely involved in this type of planning and goalsetting.

Ethical Conduct. In dietetics, the *Code of Ethics for the Profession of Dietetics* is the guiding document to ethical practice. In any institution, the manager/leader assists in developing organization practices and policies that promote ethical practice. Such practices and policies will be established in purchasing, financial management, patient care issues, and information provided patients and clients, among others—and, the manager/leader sets the example for ethical behavior and integrity built on openness and trust.

Managing Change. Change occurs when there is dissatisfaction with events as they are and there is a desire to make them different. Change may occur slowly or rapidly as in the event of sudden or unplanned circumstances. The leader who welcomes change and uses it to motivate and improve a department or unit's functions will be the most successful. When all members of a unit work together to make changes, the efforts are usually rewarded by acceptance of the new procedure by all those affected. In contrast, if change is imposed by the leader, there is often resistance and slow acceptance.

Dietitians who counsel clients to make changes do not always meet with success.[22] Time constraints and client expectations that are different from the dietitian's are factors in the change process. Change models that take into consideration the complexities of behavior and one's approach to what it takes to help people change are often helpful. One approach described as helpful is the use of goal setting in a way that the client being counseled is a part of the process and understands the expected outcome.[23] A model for goal setting is shown in Figure 11–2.

Recognition of the need for change by identifying the problem is the first step. One or more achievable goals for overcoming the problem will be set in the second step of the process, followed by actions toward achieving the goals. In this step, persons typically mobilize their personal and social resources and identify barriers to reaching the goal. Self-monitoring provides additional motivation to successfully attain the goal with a reward. The reward may be external, but the more effective reward is usually the internal or learning that leads to sustained performance and possible further goal setting.

Dietetics professionals constantly face change because of new developments in health care, organizational changes, and shifts in management with new mission and vision goals; even environmental or political situations create change. When changes are viewed as opportunities, they will more likely have positive results. The creative manager/leader helps create an atmosphere that welcomes and plans for this outcome.

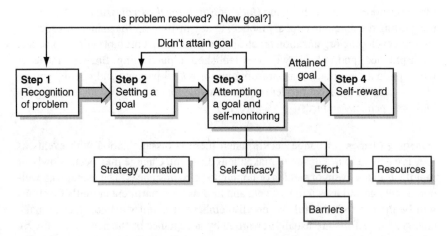

Figure 11–2   The Goal-Setting Process. *Source:* Cullen, K.W., T. Baranowski, and S.P. Smith. "Using Goal Setting as a Strategy for Dietary Behavior Change," *J Am Diet Assoc* 94, no. 12(1994): 1381–1384.

Management in Clinical Dietetics. In a 1994 survey, it was found that clinical dietitians perform a variety of management tasks in their practice settings.[24] Management is a viable component of clinical dietitians' responsibility, and knowledge of such activities helps make them competitive in the professional job market. In addition, management is often the pathway to upward career mobility. With the current drive for cost-effective, quality patient care, clinical dietitians are expected to exhibit management skills.

FURTHER MANAGEMENT ROLES

A noted management expert and author, Mintzberg, described a manager's job in terms of roles and behaviors. He describes the three categories, of interpersonal, informational, and decisional, shown in Table 11–3, that illustrate his top 10

Table 11–3   Mintzberg's 10 Managerial Roles

Managerial Role	Behavior
Interpersonal	
Figurehead	Represents the organization on formal ceremonial occasions
Liaison	Interacts with peers in the organization, other colleagues, and people outside the vertical chain of command to gain favors and gather information
Leader	Motivates and guides staff
Informational	
Monitor	Scans the environment for information, asks for information from subordinates and peers, and receives unsolicited information
Disseminator	Transmits information into the organization
Spokesperson	Sends information into the external environment
Decisional	
Entrepreneur	Initiates change to improve the unit and to adapt to a changing environment
Disturbance handler	Takes charge when the organization is threatened and when there is conflict and pressure beyond the manager's control
Resource allocator	Decides where the organization will expend its efforts
Negotiator	Deals with situations in which the manager feels compelled to enter negotiations on behalf of the organization

Source: Barker, A.N., M.B.F. Arensberg, and M.R. Schillen. *Leadership in Dietetics: Achieving a Vision for the Future.* Chicago: The American Dietetic Association, 1994, p. 55.

managerial roles. The ten roles are thought to be common to the work of all managers. However, the roles overlap and may gain in importance depending on the content and purposes of the manager's work. *Interpersonal* roles are a part of the formal authority of the manager and because of many interpersonal interactions, the *informational* role is critical. By using the information gathered from the interpersonal and informational roles, the manager is central in making decisions for the organizational unit.

SUMMARY

Managers and leaders possess many characteristics that are similar, but it is possible to be one and not the other. The skillful manager possesses human, technical, and conceptual abilities that permit him or her to accomplish work through subordinates and to attain goals. The leader may perform some or all of these same functions but will also inspire, motivate, and create a sense of unity and purpose. The dietitian, irregardless of area of practice, must perform management functions such as goal setting, communicating, team building, and managing resources.

DEFINITIONS

Benchmarking. Comparing performance with others for the development of better methods and procedures.

Coaching. The process by which a teacher or guide inspires and motivates.

Leadership. Qualities that allow an individual to influence the actions of others.

Management. The activities involved in the functions of an organization.

Mentoring. Teaching and guiding by instructing, demonstrating, encouraging, and role modeling.

Resource Management. The handling of money, equipment and supplies, or personnel essential to the administration of an organizational unit.

Strategic Planning. Long-range planning that involves data gathering, data analysis, development of goals and objectives, and action plans.

REFERENCES

1. Covey, S.R. *Principle-Centered Leadership.* New York: Simon and Schuster, 1990, p. 184.

2. Drucker, P.F. *Managing for the Future: The 1990s and Beyond.* New York: Ruman Talley Books/Plume, 1992.

3. Ibid.

4. Barker, A.N., M.B.F. Arensberg, and M.R. Schiller. *Leadership in Dietetics: Achieving a Vision for the Future.* Chicago: The American Dietetic Association, 1994.

5. Jackson, R. *Nutrition and Food Services for Integrated Health Care: A Handbook for Leaders.* Gaithersburg, MD: Aspen Publishers, 1997.

6. See Note 2.

7. Carter, D.D., and M.F. Nettles. "Dietitions as Multidepartment Managers in Health Care Settings." *J Am Diet Assoc* 103(2)2003: 237–240.

8. Brown, D. "Ways Dietitians of Different Generations Can Work Together." *J Am Diet Assoc* 103, no. 11(2003): 1461–1462.

9. Chernoff, R., ed. *Communicating as Professionals,* 2nd ed. Chicago: The American Dietetic Association, 1994.

10. Holli, B.B., and R.J. Calabrese. *Communication and Education Skills: The Dietitian's Guide,* 2nd ed. Philadelphia: Lea and Febiger, 1991.

11. Michalczyk, D. "Impact Your Practice: Communicate Effectively Online." *J Am Diet Assoc* 102, no. 6(2002): 778–779; and Alessandra, T., and P. Hunsaker. *Communicating at Work.* New York: Fireside, 1993.

12. Hendricks, W. ed. *Coaching, Mentoring, and Managing.* Franklin Lakes, NJ: Career Press, 1996.

13. See Note 2.

14. "Position of the American Dietetic Association: Cost-Effectiveness of Medical Nutrition Therapy." *J Am Diet Assoc* 95, no. 1(1995): 88–91 (reaffirmed 1997 and 2004).

15. McKnight, L.E.G., M.L. Dundas, and J.T. Girvan. "Dietetics Program Directors Affirm the Importance of Teaching Financial Management Concepts in All Areas of Practice." *J Am Diet Assoc* 102, no. 2(2002): 82–84.

16. Johnson, B.C., and J. Chambers. "Foodservice Benchmarking: Practices, Attitudes, and Beliefs of Foodservice Directors." *J Am Diet Assoc* 100, no. 2(2000): 175–180.

17. See Note 4.

18. Ibid.

19. JCAH. *Accreditation Manual for Hospitals,* vol. 14, no. 5. Oakbrook Terrace, IL: Author, 1996, pp. 6–7.

20. Spears, M. *Foodservice Organization: A Managerial and Systems Approach.* Englewood Cliffs, NJ: Prentice Hall, 1995.

21. Sullivan, B.C. In Jackson, R. *Nutrition and Food Services for Integrated Health Care: A Handbook for Leaders.* Gaithersburg, MD: Aspen Publishers, 1997, pp. 108–111.

22. Laquatra, I. "A Challenge to Change the Way We Help." *J Am Diet Assoc* 102, no. 11(2001): 1318.

23. Cullen, K.W., T. Baranowski, and S.P. Smith. "Using Goal Setting as a Strategy for Dietary Behavior Change." *J Am Diet Assoc* 101, no. 5(2001): 562–565.

24. Digh, E.W., and R.P. Dowdy. "A Survey of Management Tasks Completed by Clinical Dietitians in the Practice Setting." *J Am Diet Assoc* 94, no. 12(1994): 1381–1384.
25. Mintzberg, H. "The Manager's Job: Folklore and Fact." *Harvard Business Review* (July–August 1975).

CHAPTER 12

The Dietitian as Educator

"Education is a lifelong process, an individual responsibility to be shared and used for personal growth and to benefit our customers and our community."[1]

Outline

- Introduction
- Educational Activities
- Learning to Teach
  - Theories of learning
  - Types of learning
- Designing Instruction
  - Assessment of the needs of learners
  - Performance objectives
  - Assessment instruments
  - Instructional strategy
  - Instructional materials
  - Evaluation
- Educator Roles
  - Mentor
  - Coach
  - Preceptor
  - Counselor
  - Communicator
- Types of Learning
  - Service learning
  - Problem-based learning
  - Project-based learning

- Adults as Learners
- Teaching Groups and Teams
- Summary

INTRODUCTION

Dietitians sometimes reveal that they chose dietetics as a career in part because they did not view themselves as a classroom teacher. The reality, however, is that all dietitians are educators, frequently in locations other than the classroom. The educational settings are as diverse as the careers in which dietitians work; the learners are individuals and groups of all ages. For example, the dietitian who works in clinical dietetics in a hospital or other health care center teaches patients, families, and allied health personnel. A dietitian in food service management teaches and trains food service personnel and may teach others in other departments. In community dietetics, the dietitian counsels and teaches community groups as well as individuals. Dietitians in business or private practice may teach patients, other personnel, and the public. In all areas of practice, the dietitian may also teach dietetic interns and dietetic technician students.

The educator role is one of the most important a dietitian fulfills. Knowledge of subject matter is attained by the professional through academic preparation in a degree program and practical experience in an internship. Added to this knowledge is an understanding of how to teach effectively and how people learn. Observation of other educators, continuing education, and professional experience as well as practice lead to expertise as an educator.

Dietitians need to possess several skills regardless of their position. These include verbal and nonverbal communications, public speaking, behavior modification and motivation, principles of learning, teaching methods and techniques, and knowledge about how to work with groups. These skills can be learned and improved the more they are used.

EDUCATIONAL ACTIVITIES

The Commission on Dietetic Registration conducted a dietetic practice audit of dietitians and dietetic technicians in 1995.[2] Dietitians who registered between 1986 and 1995 and a smaller group from 1969 (the start of registration) and 1985 along with a representative group of registered dietetic technicians (DTRs) were surveyed. The types of positions varied widely among both groups, but many similarities were found in the activities performed. See Table 12–1.

Table 12–1   Educational Activities Performed by the RD and DTR

Activity	Percentage Performing Activity	
	RD	*DTR*
Nutrition Education for Public Groups		
Delivers preplanned educational programs	5.3	15.0
Selects/adapts/delivers educational programs	16.4	14.8
Selects educational methodologies, develops materials, and delivers programs	29.7	11.6
Designs, manages, and coordinates programs including evaluating outcomes	15.0	3.8
Establishes goals and priorities for educational programs for organization	11.7	3.2
Total	**78.1**	**48.4**
Computer Information Systems		
Uses computer to process data in prescribed format (e.g., nutrient analysis, patient/client information, purchasing records, literature searches)	54.4	52.1
Monitors and solves problems related to the computer—generates reports	11.7	7.5
Manages computer systems for department operations	4.4	5.3
Proposes information systems redesign with consultation from computer experts	5.0	1.5
Designs information systems applications	0.8	0.2
Total	**76.3**	**66.6**
Educational Training of Health Professionals and Students		
Develops and presents seminars or lectures for health professionals or students	22.8	9.7
Acts as preceptor for dietetics or other students	35.6	22.1
Plans, develops, and implements dietetics nutrition education courses and curricula for health professionals or students	10.8	3.0
Directs a dietetic education program	1.3	0.8
Directs formal educational programs for multiple disciplines	2.2	0.7
Total	**72.7**	**36.3**
Nutrition Education and Counseling of Individuals		
Implements specific educational protocol and adapts as needed	7.8	16.2

(continues)

Table 12–1   continued

Activity	Percentage Performing Activity	
	RD	DTR
Assesses need for delivery and evaluates effect of nutrition counseling for individuals with common medical/nutritional conditions	20.8	35.2
Assesses need for, delivers, and evaluates effect of nutrition counseling for individuals with complex medical/nutritional conditions	33.5	13.1
Develops standards of care to promote optimal nutrition education/counseling	14.5	4.7
Designs and develops interdisciplinary services to meet complex health care and nutrition needs	8.2	1.5
Total	**84.8**	**70.7**

Source: Adapted from Kane, M.T., et al. "1995 Commission on Dietetic Registration Dietetics Practice Audit." *J Am Diet Assoc* 96(1996): 1292–1301.

As shown in Table 12–1, between 73 and 85 percent of registered dietitians (RDs) performed educational activities as part of their job responsibility. The most frequent activity was *nutrition education and counseling of individuals*. Among the dietetic technicians, the most frequent educational activity was also in *nutrition education and counseling of individuals*.

LEARNING TO TEACH

The success of any educational undertaking is an outcome of the planning that occurs prior to the learning session. Many dietitians have taught in-service classes or community groups with inadequate time to plan and prepare or uncertainty about how to proceed, resulting in a disappointing session for all. Inexperience, lack of information about the learner and his or her background and needs, lack of knowledge about instructional methods, and inadequate preparation are factors that can easily defeat a learning situation.

The clinical dietitian who teaches patients will find it helpful to have an understanding of teaching skills as illustrated in Table 12–2. For instance, *interpersonal* skills help build trust and rapport between the student and teacher. *Essential teaching* skills are general strategies that form a framework for most teaching. *Presentation* skills help make instruction memorable; in other words they improve the likelihood that patients will apply what they learn.[3]

Table 12–2　Effective Patient Teaching Skills

Interpersonal skills	Presentation skills
Respect for the patient	Opening
Vocal behavior	Negotiating objectives
Body language	Organizational clarity
	Stimulus variety
Essential teaching functions	Highlighting
Assessment	Active involvement
Evaluation	Using visual aids
Feedback	Use of examples
Independent practice	Closing
Adherence counseling skills	
Specifying a behavioral plan	
Negotiating the treatment plan	
Accountability and follow-up	
Use of behavioral techniques	

Source: Roach, R.R., et al. "Improving Dietitian's Teaching Skills," *J Am Diet Assoc* 92, no. 12(1992): 1466–1473.

Theories of Learning

Two major theories of learning, *behavioral and cognitive,* have been described.[4] Behaviorists concentrate on how individuals learn new habits or procedures through stimulus and response. Cognitive theorists believe that the learner becomes an active participant in the learning process and is goal directed.

Types of Learning

Education programs are based on learning outcomes or categories of learning described as *domains of learning.* One classification by Gagne describes five types of learning skills or outcomes as follows:[5]

1. Psychomotor skills. The learner acquires motor skills along with the know-how to perform tasks.
2. Intellectual skills. Information-processing skills allow the learner to perform a new activity.
3. Verbal processing skills. The learner is able to provide information through stating or listing or describing something.
4. Attitudinal skills. The learner makes choices or decisions to act in certain ways. These may be long-term goals that determine a person's ability to perform psychomotor or other skills.

5. Cognitive skills. The learner has attained abstract strategies to become self-directed through the use of intellectual skills.

DESIGNING INSTRUCTION

The steps involved in preparing to teach are shown in Figure 12–1. The steps in the process include the following:

Assessment of the Needs of Learners

In this step, the instructor finds out what individuals already know and what they need to know. This may be accomplished through tests or surveys, oral interviews, or by focus groups. At times, the need for instruction may result from a needs assessment, from practical experience with learning difficulties of earlier learners, analysis of someone performing a job, or a change in organizational needs. It is important to know the present status of persons regarding their knowledge, skills,

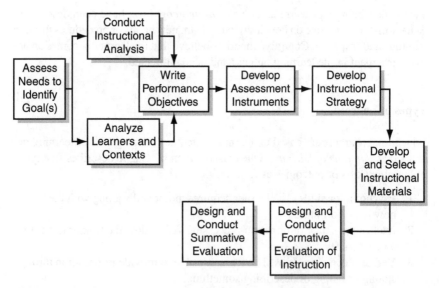

Figure 12–1   Introduction to Instructional Design. *Source:* Adapted from Dick, W., and L. Carey. *The Systematic Design of Instruction,* 4th ed. New York: Harper Collins College Publishers Inc., 1996, p. 2.

abilities, aptitudes, interests, personality, educational background, and psychological readiness to learn. It may not be possible to discern all these factors in every situation; however, this initial step is important in knowing how to plan instruction.

Performance Objectives

Based on the assessment completed in step 1, specific statements are written describing what the learner will be able to accomplish. The objectives will identify the skills to be learned, the conditions under which they are performed, and the criteria for successful performance. They need to be measurable and focused on the learner.[6]

A classification system for performance objectives often referenced by educators includes three categories or domains: *cognitive, affective, and psychomotor*. The *cognitive* domain has six categories:[7]

1. Knowledge. The acquiring and remembering of specific materials.
2. Comprehension. The ability to grasp the meaning of material.
3. Application. The ability to use learned material in new situations.
4. Analysis. The ability to break down material into its component parts for an understanding of how it is organized.
5. Synthesis. The ability to put parts together to form a new whole.
6. Evaluation. The ability to judge the value of material for a given purpose.

According to Bloom and colleagues, learning progresses from the first or lowest level (knowledge) to the highest (evaluation).[8]

The second or *affective* domain concerns changes in attitude, values, beliefs, appreciation, and interests. Krathwohl and others have developed a listing of educational objectives in the affective domain.[9] They are:

- Receiving. The learner becomes aware of and receives the lesson.
- Responding. The learner becomes involved in a subject or activity.
- Valuing. The learner believes in and accepts the value of the information.
- Organization. The learner conceptualizes and organizes a value system.
- Characterization. Values have been internalized and control behavior.

In the *psychomotor domain,* several levels are identified during which the development of manual or motor skills progresses to increasingly more difficult steps.[10]

1. Perception. The learner becomes aware of objects through the senses and selects the sensory perceptions needed to act.
2. Set. A readiness to perform tasks is demonstrated, both mentally and physically.
3. Guided response. The teacher or trainer guides the learner in an activity.

4. Mechanism. Through practice, the learner becomes proficient at the task.
5. Complex overt response. A level of skill is attained over time, or performance is characterized by accuracy and speed.
6. Adaptation/origination. Motor proficiency is altered in new situations and new physical acts based on skills attained are created or "originated."

A behavioral objective has three parts: a description of the skill or behavior identified in the analysis, a description of the conditions under which the learner carries out the task, and the criteria that will be used to evaluate learner performance.[11] An example of an objective demonstrating these parts follows:

the clinical dietitian will conduct a nutritional assessment for each patient admitted to the health care unit within 24 hours after admission and record the findings in the patient's chart.

The type of action is designated by the verb selected to demonstrate the action. Psychomotor skills are usually expressed in terms of an action verb, such as *perform*. Intellectual skills are shown by verbs such as *discriminate, identify, classify,* and *demonstrate*. Verbs that are general, such as know or understand, are too vague unless the specific behavior that demonstrates acquisition of knowledge can be described.

To decide if the objective is clear and feasible, the instructor constructs a test item to measure the learner's performance.

Assessment Instruments

The term *assessment* denotes broader activity than just testing and includes many types of activities that may be used to assess performance. When tests are used, the basic types are the pretest and the posttest. The pretest measures skills that have been identified as critical to beginning instruction and that the designer plans to develop in the instruction. If the material to be taught is new to the learner, a pretest is probably not necessary because it can be assumed they have no background knowledge or skill in the subject. The posttest should focus on the objectives. Its main purpose is to help the designer identify areas of instruction that need revision.

Several types of tests may be used, and the type is based on the objective. The chart in Table 12–3 is a guide to matching the type of behavior with related test items.

Other assessment instruments to measure performance, product, and attitudes include the following: a checklist, a rating scale that requires levels of discrimination (poor to excellent, for instance. the Likert scale), a frequency count, or a combination of formats.

Table 12–3   Type of Behavior and Related Test Item Types

	Types of Test Items						
Type of Behavior Stated in Objective	*Essay*	*Fill-in-the-Blank*	*Completion*	*Multiple Choice*	*Matching*	*Product Checklist*	*Live Performance Checklist*
State	X		X				
Identify		X	X	X	X		
Discuss	X		X				
Define	X		X				
Select				X	X		
Discriminate				X	X		
Solve	X	X	X	X		X	
Develop	X		X			X	
Locate	X	X	X	X	X	X	
Construct	X	X	X			X	X
Generate	X		X			X	X
Operate/Perform							X
Choose (attitude)	X			X			X

Source: Dick, W., and L. Carey. *The Systematic Design of Instruction,* 4th ed. New York: Harper Collins College Publishers, Inc., 1996, p. 148.

Instructional Strategy

The instructional strategy refers to the sequencing and organizing of information to be learned and deciding on the delivery format. The objectives for lower-level skills are usually the starting point, progressing to higher levels of learning. Factors to be considered include: the age level of the learners, the complexity of the material, the type of learning to take place, the activities to be included, and the amount of time required to include all the events planned. Prior to actual instruction, it is helpful to consider the motivation of the learners. Motivation involves gaining the learners' attention by asking questions, creating mental challenges, using human interest examples, and humor. Establishing the relevancy of the material for the learners and instilling confidence that they can master the material are important.

The instructor next plans the format and presentation procedures for each objective or cluster of objectives. The learning activities may differ for the cognitive, affective, and psychomotor domains. In general, the techniques used should actively involve the learner insofar as it is possible to do so.

An example showing strengths and weakness of teaching methods is shown in Table 12–4.

Job instruction training is a four-step process often used to teach skills. In the first step, the learner is prepared by putting him or her at ease, finding out what he

Table 12–4   Strengths and Weaknesses of Teaching Methods

	Strengths	Weaknesses
Lecture	Easy and efficient Conveys most information Reaches large numbers Minimum threat to learner Maximum control by instructor	Learner is passive Learning by listening Formal atmosphere May be dull, boring Not suited for higher level learning in cognitive domain Not suited for manual learning
Discussion Panel Debate Case study	More interesting, thus motivating Active participation Informal atmosphere Broadens perspectives We remember what we discuss Good for higher level cognitive, affective objectives	Learner may be unprepared Shy people may not discuss May get sidetracked More time consuming More threatening Size of group limited
Projects	More motivating Active participation Good for higher level cognitive objectives	
Laboratory experiments	Learn by experience Hands on method Active participation Good for higher level cognitive objectives	Requires space, time Group size limited
Simulation Scenarios In-basket Role playing Critical incidents	Active participation Requires critical thinking Develops problem solving skills Connects theory and practice More interesting Good for higher level cognitive objectives and affective objectives	Time consuming Group size limited
Demonstration	Realistic Appeals to several senses Can show a large group Good for psychomotor domain	Requires equipment Requires time Learner is passive, unless can practice

Source: Holli, B.B., and R.J. Calabrese. *Communication and Education Skills: The Dietitian's Guide,* 2nd ed. Philadelphia: Lea & Febiger, 1991, p. 197.

or she already knows, stating the job to be learned, and developing interest. In step 2, the material is presented and explained by stressing key points, instructing clearly and completely, illustrating and demonstrating, and then summarizing. Step 3 tests how much the learner has retained by trying out the procedure, coached by the trainer or instructor. The final step, step 4, is to let the learner proceed with supervision to ensure the task is performed accurately and consistently.

Davis describes ways to assist students as they internalize new information:[12]

1. Accept the fact that students learn, think, and process information in different ways. The differences are most noticeable when the new information is abstract and complex. Learners do not make uniform progress. Research further suggests that men and women may differ in "ways of knowing" and that women may respond better to small group and experiential learning activities.
2. Tell learners what they are expected to learn by introducing the key concepts and the more important points in one session.
3. Give a framework for new facts. Outlines, study questions, and study guides help create the framework.
4. Recognize that learners' previous knowledge influences what they learn in a new situation. Learners fit new information into their own familiar framework to give attention and organize the new material.
5. Relate material to something already meaningful, relevant, or important to the learner. Draw connections between what they already know and what they are learning.
6. Limit the amount of information presented. New information is absorbed best when presented in small amounts.
7. Broad concepts are understood and remembered and are therefore more meaningful than facts or details.
8. Provide opportunities for active learning. Students learn best by doing, writing, discussing, or taking action. Allow them to summarize, paraphrase, or generalize about the important ideas through group discussion, simulation, case studies, and written assignments.

Instructional Materials

Although this step follows the development of instructional strategy in the model (Table 12–1), it is typically performed during preparation for instruction. The selection of the best materials to use is based on the learning skills desired. If psychomotor skills are expected, specific practice equipment is needed. If attitudinal skills are to be the outcome, visual media is often selected. A model of media choices according to types of learning is shown in Figure 12–2.

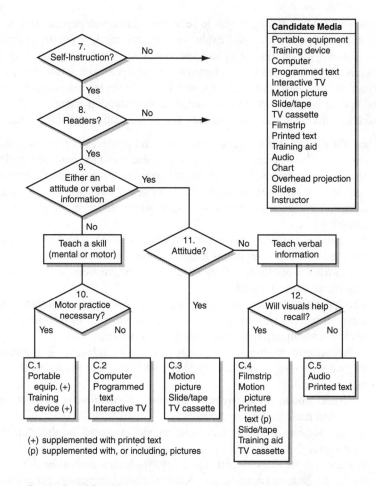

Figure 12–2   Media Selection. *Source:* Adapted from Dick, W., and L. Carey. *The Systematic Design of Instruction,* 4th ed. New York: Harper Collins College Publishers Inc., 1996, p. 2.

In choosing instructional materials, an appropriate first step is to determine if existing materials fill all or part of the needs. Such materials can be examined to determine the appropriate context, sequence, and type of information available. If a video, for instance, fills a specific need toward meeting a session's objective, excerpts of videotape, film, or pictures from the Internet might be used. Text can be scanned and made into overheads. If appropriate materials are not available, the instructor needs to develop them. If print media is predominantly used, a learner's guide will be helpful. For distance education , especially by computer, much of the instruction is learner directed and a guide is essential.

Evaluation

Evaluation shows the value or worth of an educational program. The benefits of program evaluation are:[13]

1. focuses the instructor on the objectives of the instructional program
2. provides information for decision making on all aspects of the program
3. identifies improvements in the design and delivery of learning events
4. increases application of the learning by participants
5. provides program accountability and data on the major accomplishments of the program
6. identifies ways of improving future programs

The learning objectives are the basis for evaluation. The evaluation techniques should match the focus of the objectives, such as knowledge acquisition, thinking skills, psychomotor skills or changes in attitudes, values, or feelings.

Two types of evaluation are used: *formative and summative. Formative* evaluation is the collection of data during a program. It assists the instructor to improve the instruction while it is underway. When evaluation focuses on the result or outcomes of a program, it is *summative.*

EDUCATOR ROLES

"Everything you say or do as well as everything you fail to say will communicate messages. You cannot not influence people."[14] This quote is applicable in whatever role the educator may assume because communicating through verbal interaction as well as through nonverbal cues is characteristic of all roles. Several of these roles are described in the following section.

Mentor

A mentor is a person who teaches by verbal interaction, demonstration of particular activities or skills, and role modeling. The mentoring relationship is a shared experience between a teacher and a learner. A mentor may be one's peer, an instructor, a trusted advisor, or a younger person—think of the teenager who helps a parent or a grandparent become computer literate. The mentor may also be described as a tutor in that both involve one-on-one teaching.

Mentoring has three components: internal trust and commitment from spending time together, patient leadership and time commitment, and emotional maturity.[15] In the workplace, gender or cultural differences can affect the mentoring relationship; hence the need for supervision.

Benefits shown to arise from effective mentoring include the following:[16]

- Increased job skills and job status
- Heightened awareness of organization politics and culture
- Appreciation for and use of networking
- A proactive approach to tasks and eagerness to learn
- An attitude of advocacy and willingness to tutor others

A successful statewide mentoring program for dietitians in California in 1999 resulted in positive feedback from mentors and mentees. In the program, district training was conducted using a PowerPoint lesson plan. The most meaningful outcomes included the following:[17]

- Positive feedback from those mentored
- Helping to change the direction of another person's career
- Networking and finding mentors through interactions
- The opportunity to provide support to RDs at a career crossroad
- Connection of RDs with skills and those who desire them
- Opened options that RDs may not otherwise have available
- Informal contacts with students interested in the program
- The potential to assist RDs in developing their education plans for the Professional Development 2001 certification
- The resources available to those interested in the mentoring process

Coach

A coach is one who inspires and motivates others. Coaching is sometimes described as the role assumed with individuals who are already achieving at a high level and need only a pat on the back and positive feedback for continued high performance. The coaching role is effective only when involvement and trust are created, when expectations are clarified, performance is acknowledged, actions are challenged, and achievement is rewarded.[18] The football coach is the classic example of one who performs all these functions in the expectation of having a winning team.

Coaching is similar to "reflective teaching" in that the teacher demonstrates a new procedure or piece of information and the learner listens and learns. The learner performs and the coach responds with advice, criticism, explanation, description, or further demonstration. The learner "reflects" and compares the new information to his or her previous knowledge and acts accordingly.

Preceptor

The preceptor is one who provides direction and instruction, supervises performance, and evaluates learners in applied practice. The dietitian who oversees a dietetic intern in supervised practice has the title of preceptor.[19,20] A preceptor must have good interpersonal and time management skills as well as subject matter competence as a skilled practitioner. Preceptors are essential in dietetics education and to the future of dietetic practice.

A description of the various roles as perceived by the teacher, preceptor/ teacher, preceptor, preceptor/mentor, and mentor is shown in Table 12–5.

Counselor

The role of counselor has two parts: interviewing and counseling. Interviewing involves the gathering of information that is then used to counsel a patient or a client. Counseling in a process of listening, accepting, clarifying, and helping clients form conclusions and develop plans of action. The process is guided by the dietitian toward helping individuals learn about themselves and about methods of coping with their dietary problem.[21]

Motivational interviewing has been defined as a way of helping others bring about behavior change such as curbing addictive behaviors.[22] This technique was used in a study that led to increased fruit and vegetable intake in African Americans.[23] This type of counseling is also described as a "directive, client-centered" style for eliciting behavior change by helping clients explore and resolve ambivalence.[24]

A cognitive interview technique is sometimes used to assist in understanding how audiences or individuals process information. Respondents are led through a survey or message and asked to respond with their thoughts, feelings, or ideas that come to mind. With this information, better messages are formed and valuation tools are targeted.[25]

Table 12–5   Preceptor Roles

	Teacher	Preceptor/Teacher	Preceptor	Preceptor/Mentor	Mentor
View of Intern	View intern as a student[a]		View intern as a prospective coworker[b]		View intern as a colleague[b]
Conceptual focus	Focus on discipline-based learning[b]		Focus on practice-based learning[a]		Focus on personal development[b]
Prior knowledge		Assess intern's prior content knowledge[c]		Assume intern has necessary content knowledge[b]	
Theory/practice	Teach basic subject matter[b]		Demonstrate the incorporation of theory in practice[a]		Identify unwritten workplace policies and practices[b]
Learning experiences	Arrange useful learning experiences to help intern achieve objectives[a]		Suggest useful learning experiences to help intern achieve learning objectives[a]		Encourage intern to determine learning experiences to achieve objectives[c]
Ethical concerns		Discuss potential ethical issues[c]		Identify actual ethical concerns[b]	
Strengths-weaknesses		Identify intern's strengths and weaknesses[a]		Help intern become aware of strengths and weaknesses[a]	
Progress evaluation	Provide intern with an evaluation of academic progress[c]			Provide intern with an evaluation of professional progress[a]	

Intern self-evaluation		Identify usefulness of self-evaluation[c]	Strongly encourage intern to participate in self-evaluation[c]
Role model	View yourself as an academic role model[a]	View yourself as a professional role model[a]	View yourself as a personal role model[a]
Duration of relationship		Recognize relationship with intern is limited[a]	View the relationship with the intern as indefinite[b]

Columns represent the categorical descriptions for each role. Rows represent the functions/elements that relate to the supervised practice experience. [a]Practices preceptors indicated they "frequently" execute and do not want to change. [b]Practices preceptors executed in varying degrees from frequently or occasionally to seldom/never, but do not want to change. [c]Practice preceptors believed they should do more often.

Source: Wilson, M.A. "Dietetic Preceptors Perceive Their Role to Include a Variety of Elements." *J Am Diet Assoc* 102, no. 7(2002): 969.

Patient-centered counseling facilitates change by assessing patient needs and subsequently tailoring the intervention to the patient's stage in the process of change, personal goals, and unique challenges.[26] Four steps are followed: assessment, advising, assisting, and follow-up. In step one, assessment, the dietitian-counselor asks questions to determine present behaviors. Open-ended questions are used for the best results. See Table 12–6 for an example of using questions in the dietetic practice.

Table 12–6   A Model for Open-Ended Questioning

Questions for Assessing Stage of Change and Motivation

How do you feel about your current diet?

What problems have you had because of your diet?

Have you (ever) thought about making changes in your diet?

What would you like to change about your diet now?

Why would you like to change your diet now?

What concerns do you have about changing your diet now?

What reasons might you have to want to maintain your current diet?

What would motivate you to maintain your current diet?

Questions for Assessing Past Experiences with Dietary Change

Have you ever made changes in your diet?

Have you maintained these changes? If so, for how long? If not, how long did you maintain the change?

How did you make changes in your diet? What helped?

What difficulties did you encounter? How did you handle them?

Questions about Anticipated Challenges or Barriers to Change

What could get in your way of attaining your goal?

What situations will make it hardest for you to achieve your goal?

What other situations might make it difficult for you to maintain your change?

Questions about Strategies to Cope with Challenges or Barriers to Change

What could you do when you face this challenge?

What else could you do in the face of this challenge or barrier?

Who could help you cope with this challenge? How?

What has been helpful in the past to deal with this barrier?

Questions for Goal Setting

What are you willing to change in your diet now?

When? How often will you do this?

Where will you do it?

What will you have to do in advance to ensure that you are able to make and maintain this change?

How confident are you of your ability to make and maintain this change?

Questions for Follow-Up

How did you do with your plan?

What helped you stay on target?

What difficulties did you encounter?

Questions for Assessing Lapse and Relapse

What made it difficult for you to stay with your plan?

How did you feel after that?

What else could you have done to stay on track?

What would you like to do now?

Source: Rosal, M.C. et al. "Facilitating Dietary Change: The Patient-Centered Counseling Model." *J Am Diet Assoc* 101, no. 3(2001): 333.

In step two, personalized advice is given toward helping a client make changes, referring to the earlier assessment. Assisting, in step three, involves giving motivational statements and encouragement. Goals and specific skills such as self-monitoring and other problem solving will also be discussed. In the final step, follow-up toward maintaining dietary changes will be presented. In this stage, the attainment of the earlier goals will be discussed and further help offered. Again, open-ended questions are used. An example of an interview using open-ended questions is shown in Table 12–7.

Communicator

Effective communication is very important in all areas of dietetics, and almost any job description will include the need to be able to communicate at all levels in an organization or with individuals. Professionals who develop verbal and written skills, along with listening skills, establish stronger relationships with clients, patients, and staff. An excellent guide to oral, written, and visual communications is the book *Communicating as Professionals* published by the American Dietetic Association.[27]

There are seven components of the communication process.

1. The *source* is the starting point for information exchange.
2. The *message* is the idea or information transmitted verbally or nonverbally or through other means.
3. The *channel* is the pathway for messages between the sender and the receiver.
4. The *receiver* takes in the message, assigns meaning, interprets, and responds to the message.
5. *Feedback* refers to the response from the receiver to the sender.
6. The *environment* is the context in which the message occurs, such as physical surrounding, cultural, historic, or attitudinal factors.
7. *Noise* is an aural, visual, or internal factor that can distract from the meaning of the message.

The communication methods that ensure messages are received need to be carefully selected. Professionals who provide nutrition information to the public will choose methods such as television, computer, or written words. The development of actionable dietary guidance messages is described by Borra and associates through use of focus groups and surveys of consumers.[28] In their model (Figure 12–3), the issues are defined, the message developed and assessed, then fine-tuned, and validated.

In another study to determine the best means of communicating nutrition education for elderly adults, several factors were found to be the most successful.[29]

Table 12–7   Open-Ended Interview

Nutritionist (N):   What concerns do you have about your diet? (OPEN-ENDED QUESTION)

Patient (PT):   I seem to be losing motivation to eat a low-fat diet and have skipped a couple of appointments because of time pressures at work.

N: Tell me about your work. (OPEN-ENDED QUESTION)

PT: I'm a lawyer with a large company. There is a lot of pressure to produce and bring in new clients.

N: It sounds like your work is quite stressful. (REFLECTIVE STATEMENT)

PT: Yes, but it is quite challenging, pays well, and I like going to court to try cases.

N: So, even though your work is stressful, you find it rewarding. (REFLECTIVE STATEMENT)

PT: Well, most of the time, but lately I wonder where it is all going. It's really affecting my motivation and energy to keep appointments and follow a low-fat diet.

N: What other concerns do you have about your diet? (OPEN-ENDED QUESTION)

PT: That's a good question. Actually, I used to keep a food diary that was very helpful, but I don't seem to have the motivation to continue to write things down all the time.

N: I know it is hard to think about keeping food diaries when you are feeling so much stress at work. (VALIDATING STATEMENT)

What kinds of things have you done in the past to keep a food diary? (OPEN-ENDED QUESTION)

PT: I used to keep it with me at all times, but lately I'm too tired to even think about it.

N: What other kinds of things helped you keep a food diary? (OPEN-ENDED QUESTION)

PT: Reminding myself that I eat much healthier meals when I monitor what I eat.

N: What other things have been helpful to you to keep a food diary? (OPEN-ENDED QUESTION)

PT: Going over the entire food diary at the end of the day. I used to take pride in how much I learned about nutrition and how much I had been able to improve my diet.

N: You mentioned a number of things about your work and the stress you are experiencing at work. You also spoke about having little energy or motivation to attend appointments and keep food diaries. (SUMMARY STATEMENT)

I'm optimistic about your ability to work toward your goal of staying on a low-fat diet and would like to help you attain your goal. (SUPPORTIVE STATEMENT)

What do you think might help you, little by little, to get back on track with things you used to do? (OPEN-ENDED QUESTION)

Source: Rosal, M.C. et al. "Facilitating Dietary Change: The Patient-Centered Counseling Model." *J Am Diet Assoc* 101, no. 3(2001): 334.

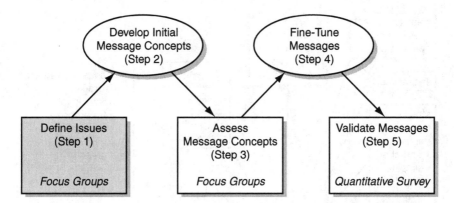

Figure 12–3   The Consumer Message Development Model. *Source:* Borra, S. et al. "Developing Actionable Dietary Guidance Messages: Dietary Fat as a Case Study," *J Am Diet Assoc* 101, no. 6k(2001): p. 679.

They included limiting educational messages to one or two; reinforcing and personalizing messages; providing hands-on activities, incentives, and cues; providing access to health professionals; and using appropriate theories of behavior change. A model was developed incorporating these elements (see Figure 12–4 on page 190).

TYPES OF LEARNING

Education through the use of methods that involve the learner in an active, participatory way can lead to very effective outcomes. Internships are examples of one type: service learning. Problem-based learning (PBL) in which a student discovers new knowledge through individual effort and project-based learning, similar to problem-based, are examples of learner involvement guided by an instructor. These three types are described in the following section.

Service Learning

This is a type of educational experience that combines explicit academic learning with community service.[30] In many professions, the idea of combining classroom study and community learning experiences is thought to enhance and retain learning. In dietetics, the internship is an example of service learning in that it combines practice with instruction. Another example is the college class that places students in a community site such as a school or elderly nutrition program for experiences

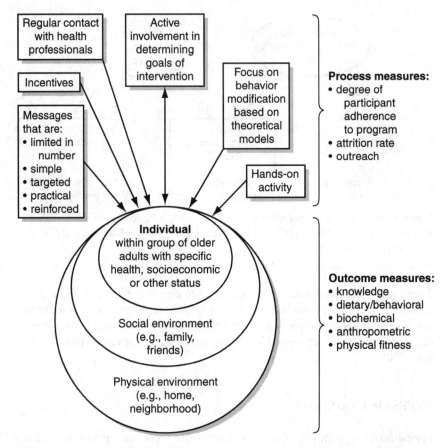

Figure 12–4   A Framework for Designing a Nutrition Education Intervention for Older Adults. *Source:* Sayhoun, N.R., C.A. Pratt, and A. Anderson. "Evaluation of Nutrition Education Interventions for Older Adults: A Proposed Framework," *J Am Diet Assoc* 104, no. 1(2004): p. 66.

that are a part of the course requirement. Seeing and experiencing nutrition applied in specific community programs makes subject matter come alive and leads to a better understanding of the value and need of community service.

Problem-Based Learning

A method used successfully in medical and business schools, this procedure is based on students working through problems to find answers to real-life situations.

PBL provides a context for students to learn critical thinking and problem-solving skills and to acquire knowledge of the essential concepts of a course of study.[31] In this method, students are presented a problem and organized into groups to discuss the problem. Students pose questions and rank the learning issues generated in the session. Students and instructor discuss the resources needed to research the learning issues. Students summarize their knowledge and connect the new concepts to older ones and define new learning issues as they progress through the problem. The benefit is that students recognize that learning is an ongoing process with continual learning issues to be explored.

The role of the instructor in PBL is to guide, probe, and support students' initiatives. When faculty incorporate PBL wholly or in part into classes, they empower students to take a responsible role in their learning. As a result, faculty must be ready to yield some authority to their students.

Project-Based Learning

Similar to PBL and case study, project-based learning is a form of instruction that places emphasis on student problem solving. It has been described as long-term problem-focused, meaningful units of instruction that integrate concepts from a number of disciplines. Both teachers and students receive support in fulfilling their roles; the teacher as facilitator and "shepherd" of projects and students by participating in a whole project as a challenge for results. A project-based learning support system has been described that supports learning through a computer-mediated interface using learner-centered software.[32] This type of learning is useful in simulations or when students have a concentrated experience such as an internship. New tools and structures are needed to support the effectiveness of this type of learning, but it provides good results amid complex and challenging projects.

ADULTS AS LEARNERS

Conducting learning sessions for adults is different than when teaching younger people. Dietitians need to be aware of the differences in order to adapt their teaching for the best learning outcomes. Holli and Calabrese describe five assumptions about adult learners as follows:[33]

1. Adults are independent and self-directed by their own preference.
2. Adults have backgrounds of experience that can be used as a resource for learning.

3. The adult's readiness to learn is based on desire to learn social roles and to solve problems. Because of this, adult employees beginning a new job would be expected to learn job expectations or an elderly patient to accept nutrition counseling for a disease condition.
4. Adult learning is oriented toward performing tasks and solving problems because adults typically have an immediate need for the information.
5. Adults are motivated by internal cues such as recognition, self-esteem, or personal satisfaction. They usually learn best when they are active participants in planning and implementing the learning experiences in which they will be involved.

TEACHING GROUPS AND TEAMS

Groups of people act in ways that are different than when they are in a one-on-one learning situation. *Group dynamics* is the term often applied to this behavior because it describes how members relate to each other, how they communicate among themselves, and how they work as a group.[34] The teacher or leader of the group needs to understand how these dynamics can affect the learning process and the way the educational message needs to be delivered.

Some of the skills to be nurtured in working with and teaching groups include the following:

1. Groups function best when all members participate and contribute ideas. The instructor can help this happen by encouraging and coaching.
2. Sharing information within the group helps to ensure that all have the same knowledge. Asking questions and initiating open discussion are ways of sharing.
3. Make sure that all members of the group understand the subject or the task. This may mean that the instructor or other group members add examples or explanations to make the information clear to all. This may also be accomplished by showing how the ideas and activities of two or more of the group are related and coordinated.
4. The instructor or leader needs to orient the group to the purpose and expected outcomes of the learning situation. Goals are clarified and direction provided that leads the discussion.
5. When verbal or other support is given for ideas and participation, the group is more likely to accept and learn. Encouraging discussion rather than debate usually leads to suggestions for new solutions and helps avoid members of the group "taking sides."
6. Recognizing that conflict and tension can arise in groups can help members and the leader be prepared to inject humor or take other means to reduce tension. A time-out or a temporary change of subject may accomplish this.

7. Another technique, *gatekeeping,* refers to being alert to signals that members of the group send about wanting to speak or otherwise participate. All members of the group should have an equal opportunity to be heard; at the same time, some may need to be encouraged to express themselves if they have not been an active participant.

When teams are focused as a work group, many of the same characteristics as evidenced in groups will also appear. Teams may be formed in order to accomplish more through the combined efforts and expertise of individual members. Participation in teams, however, requires that members understand their role and the expectations for the group.

When teams are first formed, members may be uncertain of their role and will depend on a leader to guide them into a team role. There may be conflict as team members clarify the team's goals. The leader then needs to redirect the energies of the team by encouraging open communication. As relationships become cohesive, the team becomes a functioning unit and develops patterns of communication and behavior. The leader facilitates decision making and problem solving. The team members find ways of handling conflict, and ways therefore develop that become standards for evaluating team performance. Finally, the team prepares for a change, a regrouping, a change in leader, or a change in the goals for which the group was formed.

SUMMARY

The role of educator is one of the most important of all those performed by the dietitian and dietetic technician. To be an effective educational leader, the professional must have a working knowledge of the education process of assessing learners' state of knowledge, setting learning goals, planning learning content and delivery methods, and evaluating the outcomes of the learning.

The dietitian may function in a number of educator roles as a mentor, a coach, a preceptor, or a counselor. The effective teacher in any of these roles is skilled in communications and has the qualities of a leader in understanding individuals and groups and fostering productive working relationships.

DEFINITIONS

Assessment. The process of valuating actions or conditions on which to base further activity.

Cognitive Skills. The application of intellectual capabilities to accomplish objectives.

Domain of Learning. A group or category of ideas, learning strategies, or classification system.

Education. The systematic instruction and training designed to impart knowledge and develop a skill.

Instruction. The activity by which knowledge or teaching is imparted.

Practitioner. One who performs in an area of practice or position.

Psychomotor Skills. The ability to perform physical tasks based on knowing or thinking.

Supervision. The process of directing the work, workers, or the operation of an organization.

Training. Actions by which person are brought to a desired standard of efficiency or behavior by instruction and practice.

REFERENCES

1. Puckett, R.P. "Education and the Dietetics Profession." *J Am Diet Assoc* 97, no. 3(1997): 252–353.

2. Kane, M.T., A.S. Cohen, E.R. Smith, C. Lewis, and C. Reidy. "1995 Commission on Dietetic Registration Dietetics Practice Audit." *J Am Diet Assoc* 96(1996): 1292–1301.

3. Roach, R.R., J.W. Pichert, B.A. Stetson, R.A. Lorenz, E.J. Boswell, and D.G. Schlundt. "Improving Dietitian's Teaching Skills." *J Am Diet Assoc* 92, no. 12(1992): 1466–1473.

4. Holli, B.B., and R.J. Calabrese. *Communication and Education Skills: The Dietitian's Guide,* 2nd ed. Philadelphia: Lea and Febiger, 1991.

5. Gagne, R.M. *Instructional Technology: Foundations.* Hillsdale, NJ: Lawrence Erlbaum Associates, 1987.

6. Mager, R.F. *Preparing Instructional Objectives,* 2nd ed. Belmont, CA: David S. Lake Publisher, 1984.

7. Bloom, B.S., M. Engelhard, E. Furet, W. Hill, and D. Krathwohl. *Taxonomy of Educational Objectives. Handbook 1: Cognitive Domain.* New York: David McKay, 1956.

8. Ibid.

9. Krathwohl, D., B.S. Bloom, and B. Masia. *Taxonomy of Educational Objectives. Handbook II: Affective Domain.* New York: David McKay, 1964.

10. Simpson, E. "The Classification of Educational Objectives in the Psychomotor Domain." *Illinois Teacher of Home Economics* 10(1966): 110.

11. See Note 5.

12. Davis, B.G. *Tools for Teaching.* San Francisco: Jossey-Bass, 1993.

13. Caffarelli, R.S. *Planning Programs for Adult Learners.* San Francisco: Jossey-Bass, 1994.

14. Hendricks, W., ed. *Coaching, Mentoring and Managing.* Franklin Lakes, NJ: Career Press, 1996.

15. Kaye, B, and B. Jacobson. "Reframing Mentoring." *Training and Development* 50(1996): 44–47.

16. See Note 14.

17. Schatz, P.E., T.J. Bush-Zurn, C. Aresa, and K.C. Freeman. "California's Professional Mentoring Program: How to Develop a Statewide Mentoring Program." *J Am Diet Assoc* 103, no. 1(2003): 73–76.

18. See Note 14.

19. Marincic, P.Z., and E.E. Francfort. "Supervised Practice Preceptors' Perceptions of Rewards, Benefits, Support, and Commitment to the Preceptor Role." *J Am Diet Assoc* 102, no. 4(2002): 543–545.

20. Hoffman, J.A. "Benefits Associated with Serving as a Preceptor for Dietetic Interns." *J Am Diet Assoc* 100(2000): 1195–1197.

21. See Note 3.

22. Thorpe, M. "Motivational Interviewing and Dietary Behavior Change." *J Am Diet Assoc* 103, no. 2(2003): 150–151.

23. Resnicow, K., A. Jackson, T. Wang, F. McCarty, W.W. Dudley, and T. Baranowski. "A Motivational Interviewing Intervention to Increase Fruit and Vegetable Intake Through Black Churches: Results of the Eat for Life Trial." *Am J Pub Health* 91(2001): 1686–1693.

24. See Note 21.

25. Carbone, E.T., M.K. Campbell, and L. Honess-Morreal. "Use of Cognitive Interview Techniques in the Development of Nutrition Surveys and Interactive Messages for Low-income Populations." *J Am Diet Assoc* 102, no. 5(2002): 690–696.

26. Rosal, M.C., C.B. Ebbeling, I. Lofgren, J.K. Ockene, I.S. Ockene, and J.R. Hebert. "Facilitating Dietary Change: The Patient-Centered Counseling Model." *J Am Diet Assoc* 101, no. 3(2001): 332–341.

27. Chenoff, R. ed. *Communicating as Professionals,* 2nd ed. Chicago: American Dietetic Association, 1994.

28. Borra, S., L. Kelly, M. Tuttle, and K. Neville. "Developing Actionable Dietary Guidance Messages: Dietary Fat as a Case Study." *J Am Diet Assoc* 101, no. 6k(2001): 678–684.

29. Sayhoun, N.R., C.A. Pratt, and A. Anderson. "Evaluation of Nutrition Education Interventions for Older Adults: A Proposed Framework." *J Am Diet Assoc* 104, no. 1(2004): 58–69.

30. Kim, Y., and A. Canfield. "How to Develop a Service Learning Program in Dietetics Education." *J Am Diet Assoc* 102, no. 2(2002): 174–176.

31. Dietetic Educators of Practitioners Practice Group. "Problem-Based Learning: Preparing Students to Succeed in the 21st Century," *DEP Line* 17, no. 3(1998): 1–5.

32. Laffey, J., T. Tupper, D. Musser, and J. Wedman. "A Computer-Mediated Support for Project-Based Learning." *Technology Research and Development* 46, no. 1(1998): 73–86.

33. See Note 4.

34. See Note 4.

CHAPTER 13

Research in Dietetics

"As a profession, the one thing we can predict is that the greatest changes in our practice will be the change in knowledge and how we integrate new science into our daily practice."[1]

Outline

- Introduction
- Importance of Research in Dietetics
- ADA Research Philosophy
- ADA Research Priorities
- Research Applications
- Career Opportunities in Research
  — Academic health centers
  — Food companies
  — Industry
  — Government
- Nutrition Research Centers
- Community and Public Health Research
- Research Activities of Dietitians
- Summary

INTRODUCTION

Much of the research in nutrition and dietetics is conducted by students and faculty members at colleges and universities. Some of these researchers are registered dietitians; others are food or nutrition scientists. Most faculty members are in research as well as teaching as part of their faculty responsibilities. They may conduct laboratory research such as metabolic studies in human nutrient requirements or in food science to determine utilization of specific food components. Other studies may be conducted in controlled working environments as, for example, in food service management productivity studies. Other kinds of research may deal with applied studies in nutrition education and data collection through surveys.

IMPORTANCE OF RESEARCH IN DIETETICS

"Well-designed and well-conducted research is critical for our profession, as it produces the scientific evidence upon which dietetics practice is based."[2] Any profession needs to continually reshape itself to meet ever-changing needs in society, and therefore research is essential for advancement in the profession. Not only do dietitians need to engage in research to uncover new knowledge and define new modes of therapy, but they also need to take a scholarly approach to everyday practice. As Parks and others have pointed out:

> To ensure that our clients receive only the very best dietetics care, we must develop aptitudes and attitudes for scholarship; question underlying assumptions to our knowledge base and to our practice; be curious about how science can be used to make us better practitioners, and have the courage to challenge the very essence of our current knowledge.[3]

Employers of dietitians or those using dietetic services want to be assured that the services they are using are supported by research. Research is the basis for education because it drives the core knowledge and competencies and is used in setting public policy. The ability to conduct and use research further allows professionals to be recognized by the public as a valued and credible source of scientifically based food and nutrition information.

ADA RESEARCH PHILOSOPHY

The research philosophy of the profession is the following:

> The ADA believes that research is the foundation of the profession, providing the basis for practice, education, and policy. Dietetics is the integration and application of principles derived from the sciences of nutrition, biochemistry, physiology, food management, and behavioral and social sciences to achieve and maintain people's health; therefore dietetics research is a dynamic collaborative and assimilative endeavor. This research is broad in scope, ranging from basic to applied practice research.[4]

The full statement and accompanying roles are shown in Table 13–1.

Table 13–1   ADA Research Philosophy Statement and Accompanying Roles

The ADA believes that research is the foundation of the profession, providing the basis for practice, education, and policy.

Dietetics is the integration and application of principles derived from the sciences of nutrition, biochemistry, physiology, food management, and behavioral and social sciences to achieve and maintain people's health; therefore, dietetics research is a dynamic collaborative and assimilative endeavor. This research is broad in scope, ranging from basic to applied practice research.

Dietetics professionals are responsible for incorporating research into all areas of practice. Both the Code of Ethics and Standards of Professional Practice identify the roles of dietetics professionals in research. The Code of Ethics states that the dietetics professional practices are based on scientific principles and current information. The Standards of Professional Practice state that each dietetics professional effectively applies, participates in, or generates research to enhance practice.

The Association uses research as the basis of decisions, policy, and communication in a variety of roles. The Association's organizational roles related to research include advocating, facilitating, convening, funding, disseminating, and educating its members. The Association accomplishes these roles collaboratively with other scientists and organizations. The following is an explanation of these various research roles:

Advocate   Involves identifying federal and nongovernmental agencies/organizations/ individuals who can support the Association's research agenda. Examples of the Association's advocacy roles are identifying research questions for the USDA/ERS or the Robert Wood Johnson Foundation or testifying before congressional leaders on the importance of research funding for data collection and nutrition monitoring.

Facilitator   Involves targeting key research questions to be answered and facilitating a successful process to answer these questions. For example, the ADA would facilitate partnerships or multidisciplinary collaboration between various researchers to find potential funding sources and conduct the research.

Convener   Involves convening key scientists and practitioners from various disciplines to explore new approaches in solving dietetics-related research questions. Examples might be convening a meeting to discuss research needed to address childhood weight management treatment and prevention.

Funder   Prepares, disseminates, and funds research proposals on key research questions important to the profession. Sometimes this process involves funding for research under the RFA or RFP, and other times the research is actually conducted in-house. The amount of funding is dependent on the availability of internal and external funds.

Educator   Develops professional development opportunities for members to enhance their knowledge of how to read, interpret, translate, integrate, and use research. The Association also provides professional development opportunities for members to enhance their abilities to conduct high-quality research.

Disseminator   Distributes research results to members and the public through publications, Web sites, and print and electronic media.

Source: Manore, M.M., and E.F. Myers. "Research and the Dietetics Profession: Making a Bigger Impact," *J Am Diet Assoc* 103, no. 1(2003): 111.

ADA RESEARCH PRIORITIES

The House of Delegates of the American Dietetic Association (ADA) reinforces the importance of research and passed a motion in 2001 recognizing research-related needs as follows:[5]

- Critical evaluation of research in preparation of evidence-based practice guides
- Integrating research findings into the daily practice setting
- Dietitians participate in research in the practice setting

Several guiding principles were also adopted at this time in recognition of research needs in the profession:[6]

- Current research where there is scientific consensus must be translated into practice in all settings.
- Research guides evidence-based practice.
- Positive outcomes may impact reimbursements.
- Positive outcomes affect legislation and regulations.
- There will be increased need for broader dissemination and implementation of research findings.

To support research, the ADA Foundation initiated the Research Endowment Fund to provide seed grant monies to explore research questions important to the profession.

The Committee on Research developed a philosophy statement and a diagram of ADA research roles. See Figure 13–1 for this diagram.

The research diagram illustrates how professionals integrate research into their practice. Not every type of research is included, but the major sources of research information are shown.

Research priorities for the association are delineated by the Committee on Research of the ADA. They include:[7]

1. Identify the effectiveness of methods, programs, and strategies for the prevention and treatment of obesity and associated chronic diseases and how dietitians collaborate with other health care professionals.
2. Identify the most effective nutrition and lifestyle education, communication, and behavior change strategies for positive nutrition and health outcomes.
3. Examine methods for translating existing research into effective nutrition interventions and programs. (Translational research is taking discovered facts and determining how to apply these findings to improve health and make life better.)
4. Identify effective nutrition indicators of disease risk, new methods for nutrition assessment, and appropriate health outcome measures and indicators for individuals and populations in various settings.

Research: Foundation of the Dietetics Profession
The American Dietetic Association believes that research is the foundation of the profession, providing the basis for practice, education, and policy.

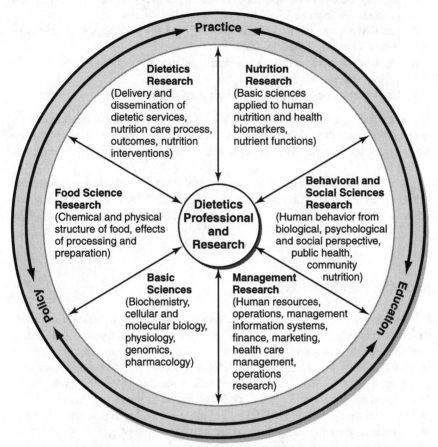

Dietetics is the integration and application of principles derived from the science of nutrition, biochemistry, physiology, food management, and behavioral and social sciences to achieve and maintain people's health.

Scientists from many disciplines contribute to the categories of research used by the dietetics professional. Descriptors of each category of research found in the wedges are for illustrative purposes and not intended to be limiting, as there are other emerging areas of research.

Figure 13–1   ADA Research Philosophy and Diagram. *Source:* Manore, M.M., and E.F. Myers. "Research and the Dietetics Profession: Making a Bigger Impact," *J Am Diet Assoc* 103, no. 1(2003): 111.

5. Identify the best methods for attracting, educating, and retaining competent dietetics professionals.
6. Identify the most effective methods for the delivery of dietetic services and payment for those services.
7. Identify ways to improve access to a safe and adequate food supply regardless of social and financial status.
8. Identify effective methods to measure and monitor customer satisfaction in various practice settings.
9. Explore the interaction among whole diet, nutrients, and gene expression.

These priorities guide decisions in the ADA about research directions and the use of resources. They provide a blueprint for the ADA's research and advocacy activities in nutrition, behavioral and social, management, basic, and food sciences areas of dietetics.

For information about types of research and research methodology, an excellent resource is *Research: Successful Approaches* by E. Monsen.[8] The reader is also referred to the many research articles regularly published in the *Journal of the American Dietetic Association*.

RESEARCH APPLICATIONS

Evidence-based dietetics practice in nutrition care is based on nutrition recommendations that translate research data and clinically applicable evidence into nutrition care.[9] This evidence-based type of research requires clinical skill, allowing the professional to apply a working knowledge of evidence to the treatment of patients. Using such evidence takes into account individual circumstances, preferences, and cultural and ethnic differences and involvement of the patient in the decision making. ADA has developed helpful guides for evidence-based practice.[10] The emphasis on this type of research is reflected in the research priorities. An overview of the evidence-based process is shown in Figure 13–2.

Outcomes research is increasingly important in the linkage of practice and research in order to make advancements in all areas of dietetics. Surveys show that while dietitians consider research important and are interested in research, many experience obstacles to performing outcomes research because of lack of research knowledge and skills, along with lack of time and money.[11,12] Eck and colleagues proposed a model for incorporating outcomes research in clinical dietetics[13] (see Figure 13–3). Hayes and Peterson advocate a training curriculum to enhance professionals' understanding of research.[14]

Trostler and Myers propose the formation of professional alliances and research-based networks within and between the national and international dietetics profession and with other health professionals as a way to improve dietetics professionals'

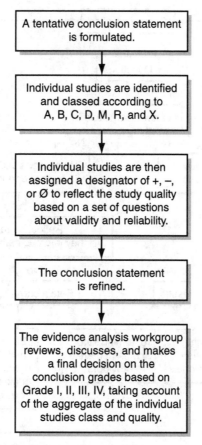

Figure 13–2 Evidence Analysis Process Overview. *Source:* Myers, E.F., E. Pritchett, and E.Q. Johnson. "Evidence-Based Practice Versus Protocols: What's the Difference?" *J Am Diet Assoc* 101, no. 9(2001): 1085.

research activity, promote dialogue, and exchange knowledge and innovative ideas.[15]

In 2003, the research committee of the ADA appointed a working group to evaluate the feasibility of forming a dietetics practice-based research group (PBRN). Such networks are formed for the purpose of enhancing research through the collaborative efforts of several practitioners to conduct research in specific problem areas and to produce outcomes that may be applied in practice. Because many practitioners lack the time or expertise to conduct research on their own, the PBRN presents an opportunity for dietetics professionals to participate in research.[16]

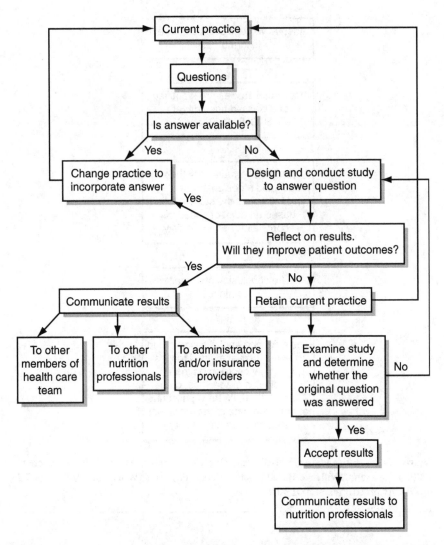

Figure 13–3 Detailed Progression of How Research and Clinical Practice Are Integrated. *Source:* Eck, L.H., et al. "A Model for Making Outcomes Research Standards Practice in Clinical Dietitians." *J Am Diet Assoc* 98, no. 4(1998): 455.

CAREER OPPORTUNITIES IN RESEARCH

Academic Health Centers

Many university-affiliated hospitals have centers dedicated to types of clinical research. Others have long-term multidisciplinary research projects that include a nutrition component. Some dietitians work at a general clinical research center (GCRC), usually associated with an academic medical center and funded by federal funds. There are 78 GCRCs funded by the National Institutes of Health (NIH) located at universities such as Ohio State, Emory, Stanford, Rockefeller, and Iowa. Research dietitians may oversee the metabolic kitchen associated with the GCRCs, analyze nutrient intakes, conduct calorimetry studies, assist in development of nutrition-related protocols, and participate in rounds and seminars.

Some GCRC dietitians manage their own research programs and direct clinical nutrition research and collaborate with the medical school faculty in research, for example, in diabetes, cancer, and acquired immune deficiency syndrome (AIDS). In recent years, several medical centers signed on to participate in long-term studies related to the NIH Women's Health Initiative. Some of these studies are designed to explore the relationship between diet and heart disease, osteoporosis, or cancer. Because each site enrolls large numbers of women, there are numerous opportunities for dietitians to become involved as nutrition counselors, data managers, or project directors.

Nutrition research sometimes involves the use of computerized nutrient databases for functional analysis, and dietitians who are adept at computers are in demand at such sites.

The need for dietitians in clinical research continues. The best dietetics practice must be based on scientific principles and sound theory. However, there is little evidence to support the value of many approaches to clinical dietetics. Additional knowledge is needed in areas of nutritional status of individuals and populations at risk for disease, identification of nutrient requirements associated with disease conditions, and nutrition interventions as therapy for disease conditions.[17] With the current crisis in health care delivery, the outcomes of nutrition intervention are an important area of investigation.

Food Companies

Many food companies employ dietitians. Roles vary but often include research related to product or recipe development. Roles can also focus on translation of research into meaningful information for the public or development of nutrition education for children, adults, and professionals.

Industry

Companies that manufacture infant formulas and medical nutritional products often employ dietitians to conduct research or to monitor clinical investigations in hospitals, nursing homes, and home care settings. Roles might include work related to:

• Nutritional needs of infants, children, and the elderly
• Acceptability of flavors and textures of products designed for oral use
• Coordination of studies to determine the effectiveness of new products
• Initiation of outcomes research to explore the cost-effectiveness of medical nutrition therapy

Government

There are many opportunities for research dietitians in government-sponsored centers and laboratories. These include positions such as:

• Nutrition scientist at the U.S. Department of Agriculture laboratory in North Dakota devoted to the study of vitamins and minerals.
• Researcher at the U.S. Army Natick Research, Development, and Engineering Center in Massachusetts involved in studies related to food behaviors and the acceptance and consumption of military rations.
• Nutrition epidemiologist at the Centers for Disease Control in Atlanta exploring patterns of nutrition-related diseases throughout the country.
• Extension specialist at a land-grant university exploring ways to maximize food production, quality, and safety.
• Life science specialist at the Congressional Research Service in the Library of Congress, answering questions and conducting research for members of Congress and staff on food safety and nutrition issues.

NUTRITION RESEARCH CENTERS

GCRCs associated with an academic medical center were described in Chapter 10. Some GCRC dietitians manage their own research programs, direct clinical nutrition research, and collaborate with the medical school faculty in research, for example, in diabetes, cancer, and AIDS. In recent years, several medical centers signed on to participate in long-term studies related to the National Institute's Women's Health Initiative. Some of these studies are designed to explore the relationship between diet and heart disease, osteoporosis, or cancer. Because each center enrolls large numbers of women, there are numerous opportunities for dietitians to become involved as nutrition counselors, data managers, or project directors.

The Agricultural Research Service of the U.S. Department funds six Human Nutrition Research Centers, which are associated with academic health centers and universities. These include the Children's Nutrition Research Center at Baylor College of Medicine in Houston the Arkansas Children's Nutrition Center at Arkansas Children's Hospital and the University of Arkansas for Medical Sciences. The center at Boston specializes in nutrition research for the aging population and is associated with Tufts University. Located on the campus of the University of California at Davis, the Western Human Nutrition Research Center is concentrating on nutrition intervention strategies. The center at Beltsville, Maryland conducts basic and applied research on nutrient composition, national dietary surveys, nutrient requirements, function of physiochemicals, and similar studies. The sixth center, located in Grand Forks, North Dakota, is associated with the University of North Dakota and has research interest in mineral requirements and utilization, as well as community-based research with Native Americans.

In addition, the Cooperative Research, Extension and Education unit of the U.S. Department of Agriculture participates and funds numerous human nutrition research studies through competitive grants and in conjunction with land grant universities.

The NIH in Bethesda, Maryland supports biomedical and behavioral research domestically and abroad, conducts research in its own laboratories and clinics, and trains young researchers. The research areas in the nutrition-related areas include: aging; alcohol abuse and alcoholism; allergy and infectious diseases; arthritis and musculoskeletal and skin diseases; child health and human development; complementary and alternative medicine; diabetes and digestive and kidney diseases; and heart, lung, and blood diseases.

COMMUNITY AND PUBLIC HEALTH RESEARCH

Since the leading causes of death in the United States continue to be nutrition-related chronic diseases, more efforts and opportunities are arising in community- and population-based nutrition research. As consumers become more aware of disease consequences of their food choices and eating behaviors, they demand more evidence of science-based causes and effects. Many dietitians who previously worked only in service program areas in community and public health are seizing the opportunity for research activities that document the value of nutrition and the dietitians' role in interventions.

Schools are becoming involved in research especially suited for nutrition, healthy behaviors, and weight maintenance by providing researchers access to students that they can follow over time. Dietitians will be needed in greater numbers for these research and education programs to be successful.

Many land grant universities are conducting nutrition research in developing countries around the world. This may involve food and agriculture production, economic development, and nutritional assessment and intervention in various populations. As more and more globalization occurs, these ventures will increase, thus providing ever greater opportunities for dietitians in research.

RESEARCH ACTIVITIES OF DIETITIANS

A survey of dietitians involved in research was conducted in 2002 because it was recognized that comprehensive data about present activities of dietitians were lacking. A representative sample of dietitians was therefore surveyed.[18] The primary areas of expertise of the respondents are shown in Table 13–2.

From the study, it is obvious that dietetics professionals are involved in research primarily in behavioral and social sciences. Dietitians in academia represented the primary employment area as one would expect. As a result of the survey, both internal and external as well as future recommendations for research were developed. The study will provide direction for the future of the profession.

SUMMARY

Dietitian researchers may be based in specialized clinical research centers, government agencies, industry, or universities. Roles vary according to the employing institution's mission and purpose. Key areas of investigation relate to nutrient requirements, food and specialized nutritional products, nutrient utilization, and outcomes of medical nutrition therapy. Opportunities for participating in outcomes research in order to enhance practice exist through collaborative research that utilizes the expertise of dietitians in many practice settings.

DEFINITIONS

Academic Health Center. Hospital, medical center, or clinic affiliated with a medical school or medical residency program.

Medical Nutrition Education. Basic and applied nutrition for medical students or residents. This often requires integration of concepts related to food science, nutrition, biochemistry, physiology, pathophysiology, health promotion, and human behavior.

Table 13–2   Researchers' Primary Areas of Expertise

Areas of expertise/research category	No. responses (total=1,280)[1]
Dietetics research	
Nutrition intervention for specific disorders and nutrition support	31
Dietetics education	28
Medical nutrition therapy, outcomes research	17
Miscellaneous	41
Total	117
Nutrition research	
Nutrition, nutrition needs for specific groups	145
Nutrients, bioactive substances for disease Rx and prevention	90
Applied basic science and nutrient functions, interactions and availability	75
Nutrition biomarkers, measures	25
Total	335
Behavioral and social sciences research	
Public health, community, wellness	315
Human behavior, counseling, education	160
Epidemiology, survey methods	75
Miscellaneous	13
Total	563
Management research	
Food service food systems, management	53
Management, administration, human resource management (HRM)	35
Information systems, finance, marketing, consulting	22
Total	110
Basic sciences research	
Physiology, metabolism	60
Disease, disease pathology	25
Genomics, molecular biology	10
Miscellaneous	12
Total	107
Food science research	
Food, nutrient composition and characteristics	25
Product development, processing	10
Miscellaneous	6
Total	41
Other	
General research methods	7

(N=545 respondents; N=1,280 responses for areas of expertise[a])

[a]Multiple responses were allowed.

Source: Myers, E.F., P.L. Beyer, and C.J. Geiger. "Research Activities and Perspectives of Research Members of the American Dietetic Association." *J Am Diet Assoc* 103, no. 9(2003): 1236.

Nutrition Education. Teaching principles of normal nutrition as the basis for optimal health and disease prevention.

Outcomes Research. Studies that focus on results and application of the results of research.

Research. Systematic investigations leading to new knowledge or new applications of known information. Research may occur in numerous settings, including laboratories, schools and colleges, hospitals and clinics, libraries, worksites, nursing homes, food companies, cafeterias, grocery stores, and day care centers.

REFERENCES

1. Park, S., R. Schiller, and J. Bryk. "President's Page: Investment in our Future—The Role of Science and Scholarship in Developing Knowledge for Dietetics Practice." *J Am Diet Assoc* 94, no. 10(1994): 1159–1161.

2. Monsen, E., and L. Van Horn. "Research: The Foundation of Practice." *J Am Diet Assoc* 103, no. 7(2003): 810.

3. See Note 1.

4. Manore, M.M., and E.F. Myers. "Research and the Dietetics Profession: Making a Bigger Impact." *J Am Diet Assoc* 103, no. 1(2002): 108–112.

5. American Dietetic Association. "Priorities for Research." www.eatright.org (accessed March 13, 2004).

6. Trostler, N., and E.F. Myers. "Blending Practice and Research: Practice-Based Research Networks an Opportunity for Dietetics Professionals." *J Am Diet Assoc* 103, no. 5 (2003): 626–632.

7. See Note 5.

8. Monsen, E. *Research: Successful Approaches,* 2nd ed. Chicago: American Dietetic Association, 2004.

9. Franz, M.J. "The Lenna Francis Cooper Memorial Lecture—The Future of Clinical Dietetics: Evidence, Outcomes, and Reimbursement." *J Am Diet Assoc* 103, no. 8(2003): 977–981.

10. Vaughn, L.A., and C.K. Manning. "Meeting the Challenges of Dietetics Practice with Evidence-Based Decisions." *J Am Diet Assoc* 104, no. 2(2004): 282–284.

11. McCaffree, J. "Overcoming Obstacles to Outcomes Research." *J Am Diet Assoc* 102, no. 1(2002): 71.

12. Hayes, J.E., and C.A. Peterson. "Use of an Outcomes Research Collaborative Training Curriculum to Enhance Entry-Level Dietitians and Established Professionals' Self-Reported Understanding of Research." *J Am Diet Assoc* 103, no. 1(2003): 77–81.

13. Eck, L.H., D.L. Slawson, R.Williams, K. Smith, K. Harmon-Clayton, and D. Oliver. "A Model for Making Outcomes Research Standards Practice in Clinical Dietetics." *J Am Diet Assoc* 98, no. 4(1998): 451–457.

14. Hayes, J.E., and C.A. Peterson. "Use of an Outcomes Research Collaborative Training Curriculum to Enhance Entry-Level Dietitians and Established Professionals' Self-Reported Understanding of Research." *J Am Diet Assoc* 103, no. 1(2003): 77–81.

15. Trostler, N., and E.F. Myers. "Mainstreaming International Outcomes Research in Dietetics." *J Am Diet Assoc* 104, no. 2(2001): 279–281.

16. See Note 4.

17. Coulston, A.M. "Make a Career of Clinical Nutrition Research." *Topics in Clinical Nutrition* 10(1995): 29–33.

18. Myers, E.F., P.L. Beyer, and C.J. Geiger. "Research Activities and Perspectives of Research Members of the American Dietetic Association." *J Am Diet Assoc* 103, no. 9(2003): 1235–1243.

PART V

The Future

CHAPTER 14

The Future in Dietetics

"The dogmas of the quiet past are inadequate for the stormy present and future. As our circumstances are new, we must think anew, and act anew."[1] Abraham Lincoln

---

Outline

INTRODUCTION

As the profession progresses into the 21st century, the challenges alluded to by one of our nation's strong leaders brings a message that is true today. The new millennium brings a hypercompetitive health care environment, greatly altered by new information technologies, new business practices, new managed care and integrated health care systems, and changing consumer demands. Clearly, the dietetic profession, like all health professions, is entering a time of unprecedented volatility and change.

A growing number of driving forces will dramatically reshape the profession. Among the most significant trends are changing demographics, growing globalization, increasing consumer expectations, merging knowledge economy, technological revolution, and a restructured workforce. To be competitive in a rapidly changing environment will require an unprecedented understanding of changing health care markets, the need for developing new global competencies and capabilities, and a shift from tangible assets to an appreciation of the value of knowledge and technology. Professions aspiring to make a difference in the lives of individuals will be playing an altogether different game—competing for the future.

CHANGING DEMOGRAPHICS

Demographic factors define health care markets from three perspectives: composition, accessibility, and mobility. The two most significant demographic influences on health care delivery are the aging population and ethnic diversity. The coming years will be characterized by a rapidly increasing number of elderly who will dramatically shift the focus of health services from acute to chronic care. In addition, no change will so profoundly alter the nature of health care as the 76 million aging Baby Boomers who are interested in health promotion and disease prevention. Further, the 21st century will be characterized by growing ethnic diversity. From 1980 to 1992, the nation's Asian-American population experienced a 123 percent growth rate and the Hispanic population a 62 percent growth rate. It is predicted that within the next 10 years about 30 percent of the U.S. population will be from today's minority and racial groups and that this trend will continue.[2] (See Figure 14–1.)

Accessibility to health care will continue to be a problem. Due to high health care costs, a large percentage of the U.S. population continues to be without adequate health care. Growing poverty among the nation's rural population, ethnic groups, and at-risk elderly is not likely to improve and will place additional demands on the health care system. This gap between the "haves" and "have nots" will likely continue to broaden.[3]

A third characteristic of the U.S. health care market is mobility. Women continue to move into the workforce and are no longer available to care for aging parents.

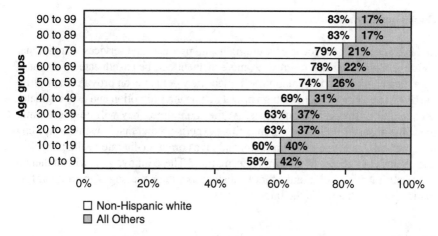

Figure 14–1 Key Trends Affecting the Dietetics Profession. *Source:* "Key Trends Affecting the Dietetics Profession and the American Dietetic Association," *J Am Diet Assoc* 102, no. 12(2002): S1823.

Extended family members have relocated to distances too far away to provide support to loved ones with acute and chronic diseases. Even those individuals within a geographic region are mobile. Of the 37 million American professionals employed outside the home, 75 percent are away from their offices at least one day a week. These individuals will buy time and convenience, along with health products and services, and will demand "on-the-go" services.

MACRO TRENDS

Globalization

As the world moves toward a global society and as free trade becomes a reality, so too should there be a free exchange of ideas and information between dietetic communities.[4] Globalization will revolutionize the current profession of dietetics. The profession will draw clients, employees, materials, and strategic partners from a single global marketplace. Many members of the profession currently lack the language skills and knowledge of cultural differences necessary to network with food and nutrition partners from around the world. Internationalization of dietetic education and practice will be a priority in the coming decade.

Consumer Expectations

In the 21st century, the focus on tailoring health products and services to individual consumers will continue to grow. A more affluent and better-educated consumer, with greater access to information, will place new demands on providers to ensure the best care. They will place a high priority on health promotion and expect greater accountability for desired outcomes. At the same time, they will be questioning the value of services. Telecommunications experts predict that new integrated circuits will become even more powerful and give computer-literate health providers and clients easy access to the same information.[5] These innovations will challenge food and nutrition communicators to distinguish their messages from misinformation, also available on the Internet.

Knowledge Economy

Over the past two millenniums, the world population has experienced a 50-fold increase. During this same time, it has been estimated that information has exploded over 250,000 times faster than the population growth. The significance of these data is often overlooked. In the dietetic profession, scientific underpinnings have provided the industry with encyclopedic amounts of new information; the application of knowledge in the practice arena has accelerated the specialized growth of the profession. To provide state-of-the art information to dietetic clients requires staying current, avoiding knowledge obsolescence, and having a commitment to lifelong learning.

Technological Revolution

Technology to produce, store, and use information will continue to expand and will dramatically change how professionals interact with clients, colleagues, and competitors. These changes in technology will, and do have, an enormous impact on health care. Although technology will be a mechanism to deliver health services and education in remote areas, it will also depersonalize care.

Information technology will affect dietetic professionals in two ways: It will remove routine tasks and allow them to become full partners on medical, management, and consumer teams and it will redefine dietetic practice roles.[6] Members of the profession will have to rethink old career assumptions, abandon obsolete practice roles, and create new opportunities. The dietetic professional of the year 2010 may work more easily to address complex health problems as information technology connects scientists, practitioners, and consumers from around the world.

Restructured Workforce

With an aging population expanding at a rate much faster than younger people, there will be fewer people to take care of the nation's health care needs. Technology may provide a partial answer. Although technology may decrease the number of traditional job openings, an entire new set of opportunities will be available to those developing computer and information management skills. Technology will also facilitate cross-disciplinary interventions and will help the profession to experiment with new types of health care teams. Interactive video conferencing, counseling, long-distance diagnostic and treatment interventions, and electronic patient records will be ways to increase access to care. This may be a partial answer to the workforce issue and help to stretch the system's resources.

CHANGING ROLES IN THE HEALTH CARE SYSTEM

In addition to these macro trends, the early 1990s brought about fundamental changes in the American health care system. Mergers, consolidations, downsizing, and outsourcing have transformed the entire way in which health services are delivered. New managed care and integrated health systems, organized along a complete continuum of care, replaced more traditional organizational structures. These systems were designed to respond to the need for cost reduction in the health care industry, to improve access to quality care, and to enhance client outcomes.

Along with challenges the dietetics profession faces as a result of the restructuring of the health industry, there are opportunities. Health care is predicted to remain one of the fastest growing sectors in the U.S. economy. For instance, by 2007, health care spending will account for about 15 percent of the nation's gross domestic product compared to the present 14 percent.[7] The growth is driven by the Baby Boomers' desire to look and feel better and the elderly's desire to live longer. In particular, trend analysts predict continued growth in the diet and fitness industry.

The other good news for the profession is that in the new market-driven health care delivery system, allied health professionals provide a cost-effective alternative to the more expensive services of physicians and nurses. To be competitive in new practice roles, allied health professionals will have to develop new roles and responsibilities. The Pew Health Professions Commission made strong recommendations about the competencies needed for these future roles: the ability to work on interdisciplinary teams; a reliance on health and information technologies, strongly grounded in science and critical thinking; and cross-functional knowledge and skills.[8] The report also suggests the emergence of new allied health professions will fall outside the sometimes rigid boundaries of currently recognized disciplines.

This movement will require innovative approaches to role definition and partnering among allied health groups.

The profession's ability to continue to deliver high-quality, cost-effective care, to enter the curative and preventive market in low-cost settings, and to systematically document the impact of nutrition interventions will determine its future.

IMPLICATIONS AND CHALLENGES FOR THE PROFESSION

The value of describing a possible future for the profession is to be able to address the challenges faced by members of the profession and to take advantage of the opportunities the future offers. Although it is admittedly difficult to predict where the profession will be with such huge changes, the questions to be asked are:

"What challenges will the future bring for the profession?"

"What new assumptions will guide planning for the future of the profession?"

"What new competencies will be needed by future professionals?"

The dietetic profession faces a number of challenges as constantly changing events and trends inevitably shape practice.

Challenge 1. Positioning dietetic professionals in an industry characterized by changing health systems. Although dietetic professionals have always focused on preventive care, they face intense competition from other health care providers, including those available via the Internet. Many health professionals are also struggling for recognition in these new health systems. The profession will need to deliver a new practitioner who brings both a multidisciplinary perspective and critical thinking skills needed to solve both client and delivery system problems.

Challenge 2. Accepting the new world of work and redefining new practice roles. Future dietetic professionals will be entering a new world of work where practice will continually change. The turbulent health care marketplace will continue to experience downsizing and dramatic restructuring, all of which affects the delivery of nutrition services. Two fundamental changes will occur: Jobs will evolve from being very narrowly defined and task oriented to more multidisciplinary and multidimensional roles; nothing will be permanent. Members of the profession will have to bring a generalist mindset to the practice area. Job flexibility will be a reality as professionals move in and out of careers and organizations many times throughout their lives.

Challenge 3. Keeping the knowledge base current and obtaining a commitment to lifelong learning. By definition, a professional is mandated to use the latest science in developing interventions and to keep practice standards current. With the rapid change in the knowledge that is brought to solve today's nutrition and eating problems, the issue of managing continuing professional education becomes a survival strategy. It has been suggested that half of what is learned as we enter the profession is obsolete within three years. This presents a tremendous need to develop lifelong learning models refocusing on professional education.

Challenge 4. Developing a sense of urgency in restructuring education for the profession. Surveys by the Commission on Dietetic Registration of dietetic practitioners and with employees indicated a need for competencies not included in dietetic programs.[9,10] At the 2000 and 2003 house of delegates meetings, a major item of discussion was dietetic education and the needs for the future. A background paper identifies several mega-issue questions regarding needs in education. A task force is developing a new plan for the future of education and credentialing for registered dietitians and registered dietetic technicians.[11] A further form of competition regarding recognition and salaries for dietetics professionals is the comparison of education levels being required for other professionals.[12] (See Table 14–1.)

Table 14–1 Entry-Level Education Requirements for Some Health Professions

Entry-Level Education Requirement	Health Professionals
Associate Degree	• Dietetic Technician, Registered • Respiratory Therapist—pursuing movement to a BS prepared clinician • Cardiovascular Technician • Registered Nurse (although there are many baccalaureate nursing degrees offered)
Baccalaureate Degree	• Registered Dietitian • Clinical Laboratory Technician • Radiology Technician—can also receive a certificate in training and/or associate degree
Advanced Degree	• Physical Therapist • Speech Pathologist • Occupational Therapist
Practice Doctorate	• PharmD • Audiologist • Dentist • Physician

Source: ADA House of Delegates. "Dietetics Education and the Needs for the Future," *HOD Backgrounder,* 2003.

Challenge 5. Keeping pace with the reengineering occurring in the industries employing dietetic professionals. Although most members are employed in health care, there will continue to be a significant number employed in the food industry. Like the health care industry, the food industry is experiencing similar downsizing, outsourcing, mergers, and acquisitions, as a result of intense competition and downturns in the economy. These changes have major implications for food and nutrition specialists, some positive and others that could be highly destructive. Continuous and overlapping change is occurring in industries and organizations in which dietetic professionals are employed, making it difficult to monitor trends shaping new practice roles.

Despite these many challenges, the profession puts together an impressive number of winning combinations. Dietetics continues to be a highly respected profession, recognized worldwide as the leading organization of food and nutrition experts. With the aging population and the maturing Baby Boomers, the demand for dietetic professionals will increase. Additionally, the industry is already a generalist profession with the capability of easily moving into multidisciplinary and multifunctional careers. Finally, the profession has a long history of encouraging the growth and development of diversity.

The profession is likely to address these changes, in part, by restructuring itself around the technology of "connectivity" and in the way its members deliver services to consumers. If downsizing and outsourcing continues in both the health care and food industries, individuals will be working in small ad hoc work groups, taking on specific tasks, and then moving on to yet another work task. Relationships will not be permanent and employee-company loyalty will not be valued.

With continuous and overlapping change in both practice settings and in interactions with others, what is brought to these new work groups will be cutting-edge knowledge. To avoid obsolescence and to keep current with the search, learning and work will occur simultaneously. Technology-based, self-directed learning will occupy a large portion of the work day. What an exciting time to be part of the dietetic profession!

COMPETITION AND COLLABORATION WITH OTHER PROFESSIONS

Competition in the future will be different from the present and past. Driven by the information revolution, the past few years have seen entirely new professions emerging and consequently new competitive products and services. Virtual "meeting and dining" rooms will allow consumers, across the nation and around the world, to meet without leaving home or work. Microrobiotics will allow a greater number of aging individuals to remain independent and in their own homes as mechanical maids "sense" and "fetch" for those unable to do so on their own. Health organizations, linked electronically, will provide access to experts around the world at the time the attending physician is in need of consultation. Digital highways will provide immediate access to the world's retail marketplace for information, programs, services, and entertainment. Technology will change the nature of competition in ways one would never expect.

There will continue to be more intensive competition among traditional sources: other health professionals, proprietary business, alternative health providers, and the media, to name a few. Challenges to the dietetics professional for nutritional services and health-related information were identified in the 2002 ADA Environmental Scan. [13] The more important question to ask, however, is "Should we be viewing these groups as competitors or collaborators?" In some cases, it will be both.

The future portends a different playing field for members of the profession. The impact of changes in the health care system has been discussed earlier. Mergers of education and information technology have produced electronic books and newsletters; personally tailored multimedia educational programs can be accessed on demand as well as interactive learning programs for at-home use. Add these with the projected mergers of telephone, television, and computer technologies, and there are unlimited capabilities to connect teachers and learners from around the world. Similarly, the food and lodging industries have opened markets in virtually every part of the world.

Probably the greatest "competitor" or "collaborator" is the rapid growth of information technology. It is the advent of the information age that is driving changes in business, government, professions, and social institutions. Future dietetic professionals will have a new set of leadership skills with a small specialty core of food, nutrition, and health. To compete, they will be experts at discovering, evaluating, and disseminating information and other resources. They will also need such futures-related leadership skills as visioning, persuasive communication, and the ability to form strategic partnerships.

COMPETENCIES OF THE FUTURE DIETETICS PROFESSIONAL

In his book, *The Knowledge Executive,* Cleveland summarizes one of the most important critical skills of future professionals in the following statement: "People who do not educate themselves, and keep re-educating themselves, to participate in the new knowledge environment will be the peasants of the information society."[14] Cleveland presents a strong case for not only understanding the power of being a "knowledge worker" in the 21st century but also for being technologically literate: being able to use existing or new technology to access and to manage the proliferation of knowledge. Others, within and external to the profession, also concur with the need for this competency.

There is general agreement among employers, educators, and practitioners that the following competencies will be needed in the future:[15]

Leadership skills—having the ability to see new opportunities, to create new opportunities, to create new visions for the profession, and to lead others through the milieu of change that will continue to be part of professional lives.

Professional and organizational awareness—understanding the mission, vision, and goals of the dietetic profession; having the ability to link food and nutrition interventions to the overall health of the individual; seeing how nutrition care fits into the goals of employment sites; appreciating organizations as dynamic political, economic, and social systems.

Problem-definition and problem-solving skills—identifying gaps between where a situation is and should be and helping others to see how to fill the gaps.

General business skills—knowing the economic impacts of food and nutrition interventions, understanding strategic management, marketing, finance, logistics, accounting, and how these business functions work together.

Team-building and interpersonal skills—because of the increasing use of outsourcing and the use of temporary personnel having strong team-building skills; similarly, having persuasive communication skills to sell new ideas and to obtain support for change.

Entrepreneurialism—having an ability to see new career opportunities, to combine that ability with necessary business skills, and to be a risk taker because of the shorter life cycles of most careers; implies a need to challenge traditional roles and prevailing approaches to delivering food and nutrition services.

Multicultural, multidiversity competence—having an openness to other cultural values, a global understanding and perspective, and the attitudes, skills, and knowledge needed to apply a global perspective to clients, colleagues, and employees' needs.

There is an urgency, voiced from many sides, that as a profession, dietitians must continue to look closely at trends and to identify those skills most critical to successful practice. Because employers are no longer hiring for today, the profession must look to tomorrow as dietitians "educate and re-educate" themselves.

CAREER STABILITY TO CAREER INNOVATION: FUTURE ROLES FOR THE PROFESSION

The future will present many new opportunities for those who assume responsibility for their own careers; for those who are entrepreneurial and willing to pursue international opportunities.

Opportunities in Health Care

The health care industry continues to grow. By 2007, health care spending will account for about 15.2 percent of the nation's gross domestic product, compared to the current 14 percent.[16] The cost of medical care for people over age 65 rises yearly as this population group grows in number. The forces behind rising health care costs are:[17]

- Advances in medical technology
- Aging
- Insufficient preventive care
- Rising government health care oversight and mandates
- Medicalization of more conditions

Because of these trends, emphasis on preventive medicine is growing.[18] Following this trend, the National Institutes of Health issues its "Healthy People" goals each decade that target specific disease conditions as well as environmental, societal, and communication needs toward improving the overall health of Americans.[19]

The demand for dietetic professionals will grow as fast as the average for all industries in the nation's economy. There will be a need for increased meals and nutrition programs in long-term care, schools, correctional institutions, residential care, community health, home health care, and health and fitness clubs, to name a few. Traditional professional roles (i.e., food service administrator or clinical practitioner) will almost become obsolete in the future. The new health care environment will see dietetic professionals managing multiple departments or providing transdisciplinary health services, in which nutrition is only part of the practice role. In the future, it will not be uncommon to see food and nutrition experts earn dual degrees in medicine, pharmacy, nursing, physical therapy, or hotel and restaurant management.

Additionally, there will be some executive-level positions in integrated health systems and in traditional health care organizations. These positions will require a new set of competencies in such areas as strategic planning, information management, marketing, finance, and cost-benefit analysis.

Edutainment

In the early 1990s, Naisbitt examined growth opportunities of greatest interest to various industries.[20] Those growth industries of greatest interest to dietetic professionals include travel and entertainment, food, health care, children's services, and the mature market. Although dietetic career opportunities in these industries may not appear readily apparent, the future entrepreneurial professional will combine educational programs and services at the same time consumers are having fun. "Edutainment" is a rapidly growing consumer trend that dietetic professionals have only begun to explore. Given the prediction of increased leisure travel, focusing opportunities around the entertainment industry could be a lucrative business venture. Cetron and Davies predict that tourism, vacationing, and travel (especially international travel) will continue to grow in the next decade.[21]

Food

Large growth in employment for dietitians in the food and food service industries is anticipated as consumer food spending by 2017 approaches a trillion dollars a year.[22] Consumers want tasty and sophisticated new foods and foods that are pure, natural, safe, and healthful. Convenience will continue to drive demand. Special food meals for segments of the population will also drive demand, especially the aging and those on weight-loss diets. The growing epidemic of obesity among children as well as adults means that dietitians with backgrounds in food science, culinary arts, food product development, and exercise and fitness are and will continue to be in demand.

The commercial food service industry will continue to provide careers for those interested in combining an interest in foods, international cuisine, and business administration. Restaurant and in-home catering will grow as consumers entertain more and cook less. Resorts hire food professionals; food manufacturers and food distributors look to members of the profession who can provide marketing support, sales training, new-product development, and food photography support. Many hotels are setting up educational/child care centers for parents traveling with kids; they need help with nutrition education programming, health and fitness programs, and developmentally appropriate feeding strategies. Associations representing health professions are also employing food and nutrition consultants to help develop transdisciplinary education programs.

Information Technology and Management

Varian predicts more information specialists will be needed in the future "to rescue managers from the proliferation of knowledge" surrounding a profession.[23] He suggests the following new career opportunities: organizers of user-friendly information on the Internet; database designers and managers; electronic writers and editors; instructional system designers; distance learning programmers and evaluators; and information entrepreneurs who can develop innovative ways for professionals and clients to connect and to work together. There will be a need for experts in such subspecialties as food and nutrition to develop, deliver, and evaluate these new and innovative educational programs. The library scientist, with a food and nutrition specialty, will be a critical future practitioner needed to organize and structure electronic data in a usable format.

Multimedia education and developing and selling electronic books, tapes, seminars, and speeches will be in great demand. Computer-related skills in any profession will translate into an average 15 percent increase in income. This gap will broaden in the future.[24] The amount of health care information accessible with information technology is increasing and the number of people with access to that information is growing. Households with a personal computer increased from 9.5 percent in 1984 to over 50 percent in 1999, and it is predicted that 70 percent of all households will own a computer by the year 2020.[25]

Research

With the advent of the information society, new opportunities will exist for those interested in the discovery of knowledge. There is a need for those interested in studying both nutrition science and nutrition intervention issues and problems.[26] New and emerging clinical protocols, intervention trials, and cost-benefit studies must be tested. Genetics and biotechnology are driving the need for discovery, too, as the effects on food and nutrition are being explored and the information made available to consumers. Similarly, there is a need for food researchers who want to develop new products or who want to understand consumer satisfaction and service quality factors; marketing research also has tremendous growth potential. Advances in the food delivery system must be modeled, simulated, and tested for quality, efficiency, cost-effectiveness, and consumer acceptance.

Private Practice

Entrepreneurialism is a guiding force in the U.S. economy and can be a way that imaginative and motivated professionals forge new areas of practice. Women start many small businesses in the United States, and this bodes well for dietetic practitioners who want to set up private practices.

The days of climbing the corporate ladder with a single company no longer exist. Creative practitioners who want to work for themselves and have more quality time with their families will find a receptive marketplace. New markets and new options are available to professionals. Entrepreneurship offers independence, expanded opportunities, and potential profits.[27, 28]

Planning for the Future

In addressing the future, dietetic practitioners must meet the challenges brought about as a result of reengineering both the health delivery system and the food industry. Those individuals who can capitalize on future trends, who understand how basic assumptions will change dietetic practice, and who proactively search out new career opportunities will be well poised for the future. Others who naively believe the future is "more of the same" will find their positions disappearing—even after many years of dedicated service.

In analyzing the future, one thing is certain—the profession must always expect the unexpected and assume the future is not an extension of the past. There are several assumptions, however, that can be made about the future that will guide people in career decision making:[29]

- The ability to connect electronically will revolutionize how, when, and where dietetic professionals will practice.
- Professionals, not the organization's management, will emerge as primary players in multidisciplinary teams; managers will become facilitators, coaches, and mentors.
- The concept of the organization will expand to include links to all external partners, including consumers.
- Most people will be connected, worldwide, forming new professional opportunities and risks.
- Services and products that dietetic professionals offer to clients will be "informationalized"; databases will be built into most products, programs, and services offered to consumers.
- Competition will no longer be limited to local, regional, or national audiences; it will be worldwide.
- Continual and just-in-time learning will be the rule for health providers and their clients.
- Most individuals will study and live with multiple cultures and languages.
- Professionals will become more entrepreneurial and innovative in their approach to career design.

As discussed, turbulent times create both threats and opportunities for members of the profession. How should individual members shape their careers to fit into future scenarios? What steps can be taken now to secure a position in the future?[30]

- Be visionary and manage your own career. Make a conscious shift of mind not to rely on traditional practice roles. Be open to future opportunities.
- Build a portfolio of skills that will position you for future career changes. There will be a need for people who can increase productivity of resources and who can develop cost-effective solutions to problems.
- If you are not techno-literate, move in that direction. Be able to design organizational and consumer programs that use multiple multimedia approaches and formats.

- Be adept at building relationships, both internal and external, to the profession. A distinct competitive advantage will come to those who know how to network and connect with consumers, experts, and information.
- Become an expert at accessing, acquiring, disseminating, and evaluating knowledge. It is the key strategic resource.
- Consider working at the periphery of the profession and related professions. Develop multi- and transdisciplinary skills. Seek out areas in nursing, physical therapy, therapeutic recreation, and medicine, to name a few, and assume personal responsibility for developing entry-level skills to add to your portfolio.
- The most critical skills that will be needed for success in the future include computer skills, statistical analyses, communication skills, an entrepreneurial outlook, financial management, critical analysis, strategic planning, negotiation, and motivation.

The entire dietetic professional infrastructure is changing. Dietitians must shift their minds individually and collectively to move with changes in the industry environment. The future belongs to those who can dream and then translate those dreams into reality.

SUMMARY

The dietetic profession is changing and becoming increasingly responsive to the needs of consumers and the marketplace. Because of changes in population demographics, increasing globalization, and changes in health care systems, the profession is faced with challenges but also great opportunities. Planning toward and preparing for the future through developing technical and personal skills such as acquisition and dissemination of knowledge, leadership qualities, and willingness to change will serve the dietitian well into the 21st century.

DEFINITIONS

Allied Health Professions. Health care organizations or groups providing services that supplement and assist those in direct health care.

Demographics. Population statistics relating to characteristics of those making up the population such as births, deaths, and ages that are used in scientific studies.

Globalization. Process of becoming worldwide in scope of business or practice.

Multicultural. Term pertaining to different cultures as among countries and populations.

Multidisciplinary. Describing a collection of several disciplines either similar or diverse in nature.

REFERENCES

1. Parks, S.C. The Future in Dietetics. In: *Dietetics: Practice and Future Trends.* Gaithersburg, MD: Aspen Publishers, 1998.

2. House of Delegates Report. "Key Trends Affecting the Dietetics Profession and the American Dietetic Association." *J Am Diet Assoc* 102, no. 12(2002): S1821–S1839.

3. *Informing the Future: Critical Issues in Health.* Washington, DC: National Academy Press, 2000.

4. Parks, S., and B. Bajus. "President's Page: Challenging the Future—An Evolving Global Perspective for the Profession." *J Am Diet Assoc* 94(1994): 782–784.

5. Cetron, M.J., and O. Davies. "Trends Shaping the Future: Economics, Societal, and Environmental Trends." *The Futurist* (January–February 2003): 27–42.

6. See Note 1.

7. *Health and Health Care 2010: The Institute for the Future.* San Francisco: Jossey-Bass Co., 2000.

8. Pew Health Professions Commission. *Critical Challenges: Revitalizing the Health Professions for the Twenty-First Century.* San Francisco: U.S.F.S. Center for Health Professions, 1995.

9. Kane, M., A. Cohen, E. Smith, and C. Lewis. "1995 Commission on Dietetic Registration Dietetics Practice Audit." *J Am Diet Assoc* 96(1996): 1292–1301.

10. Balch, G. "Employer's Perceptions of the Roles of Dietetic Practitioners: Challenges to Service and Opportunities to Thrive." *J Am Diet Assoc* 96(1996): 1301–1305.

11. American Dietetic Association House of Delegates. "Dietetics Education and the Needs for the Future." *HOD Backgrounder* (2003).

12. Ibid.

13. See Note 1.

14. Cleveland, H. *The Knowledge Executive.* New York: Truman Talley Books/EP Dutton, 1989.

15. See Note 1.

16. See Note 6.

17. See Note 2.

18. See Note 5.

19. Office of Disease Prevention and Health Promotion, "Healthy People 2010," http://www.health.gov/hpcomments/2010fctsht.htm, U.S. Department of Health and Human Services (accessed March 2004).

20. Naisbitt, J. "223 Hot, New Future Business Trends for the 1990s: A Special Report." Washington, DC: The Global Network, 1993.

21. See Note 5.

22. See Note 13.

23. Varian, H. "The Next Generation Information Manager." *Educom Review* (1997): 12–14.

24. Hansen, K., and D. Hayes. "Dietetics Professionals Online: The Way of the Web Is the Wave of the Future." *J Am Diet Assoc* 99, no. 1(1999): 1349–1350.

25. See Note 2.

26. Tuppenden, K.A. "Preparing RDs for Careers in Research? Development of a New Research Emphasis." *DEP Line* (Summer 2003): 6–7.

27. Ibid.

28. Helm, K.K. *The Entrepreneurial Dietitian,* 2nd ed. Lake Dallas, TX: K.K. Helm Press, 1991.

29. See Note 1.

30. See Note 1.

APPENDIX A

Code of Ethics for the Profession of Dietetics

(Adopted by House of Delegates of the American Dietetic Association, June 1999)

PREAMBLE

The American Dietetic Association and its credentialing agency, the Commission on Dietetic Registration, believe it is in the best interest of the profession and the public it serves to have a Code of Ethics in place that provides guidance to dietetics practitioners in their professional practice and conduct. Dietetics practitioners have voluntarily adopted a Code of Ethics to reflect the values and ethical principles guiding the dietetics profession and to outline commitments and obligations of the dietetics practitioner to client, society, self, and the profession.

The Ethics Code applies in its entirety to members of The American Dietetic Association who are Registered Dietitians (RDs) or Dietetic Technicians, Registered (DTRs). Except for sections solely dealing with the credential, the Code applies to all members of The American Dietetic Association who are not RDs or DTRs. Except for aspects solely dealing with membership, the Code applies to all RDs and DTRs who are not members of The American Dietetic Association. All of the aforementioned are referred to in the Code as "dietetics practitioners." By accepting membership in The American Dietetic Association and/or accepting and maintaining Commission on Dietetic Registration credentials, members of The American Dietetic Association and Commission on Dietetic Registration credentialed dietetics practitioners agree to abide by the Code.

PRINCIPLES

1. The dietetics practitioner conducts himself/herself with honesty, integrity, and fairness.
2. The dietetics practitioner practices dietetics based on scientific principles and current information.
3. The dietetics practitioner presents substantiated information and interprets controversial information without personal bias, recognizing that legitimate differences of opinion exist.
4. The dietetics practitioner assumes responsibility and accountability for personal competence in practice, continually striving to increase professional knowledge and skills and to apply them in practice.
5. The dietetics practitioner recognizes and exercises professional judgment within the limits of his/her qualifications and collaborates with others, seeks counsel, or makes referrals as appropriate.
6. The dietetics practitioner provides sufficient information to enable clients and others to make their own informed decisions.
7. The dietetics practitioner protects confidential information and makes full disclosure about any limitations on his/her ability to guarantee full confidentiality.
8. The dietetics practitioner provides professional services with objectivity and with respect for the unique needs and values of individuals.
9. The dietetics practitioner provides professional services in a manner that is sensitive to cultural differences and does not discriminate against others on the basis of race, ethnicity, creed, religion, disability, sex, age, sexual orientation, or national origin.
10. The dietetics practitioner does not engage in sexual harassment in connection with professional practice.
11. The dietetics practitioner provides objective evaluations of performance for employees and coworkers, candidates for employment, students, professional association memberships, awards, or scholarships. The dietetics practitioner makes all reasonable effort to avoid bias in any kind of professional evaluation of others.
12. The dietetics practitioner is alert to situations that might cause a conflict of interest or have the appearance of a conflict. The dietetics practitioner provides full disclosure when a real or potential conflict of interest arises.
13. The dietetics practitioner who wishes to inform the public and colleagues of his/her services does so by using factual information. The dietetics practitioner does not advertise in a false or misleading manner.
14. The dietetics practitioner promotes or endorses products in a manner that is neither false nor misleading.

15. The dietetics practitioner permits the use of his/her name for the purpose of certifying that dietetics services have been rendered only if he/she has provided or supervised the provision of those services.

16. The dietetics practitioner accurately presents professional qualifications and credentials.

   a. The dietetics practitioner uses Commission on Dietetic Registration awarded credentials ("RD" or "Registered Dietitian"; "DTR" or "Dietetic Technician, Registered"; "CSP" or "Certified Specialist in Pediatric Nutrition"; "CSR" or "Certified Specialist in Renal Nutrition"; and "FADA" or "Fellow of the American Dietetic Association") only when the credential is current and authorized by the Commission on Dietetic Registration. The dietetics practitioner provides accurate information and complies with all requirements of the Commission on Dietetic Registration program in which he/she is seeking initial or continued credentials from the Commission on Dietetic Registration.

   b. The dietetics practitioner is subject to disciplinary action for aiding another person in violating any Commission on Dietetic Registration requirements or aiding another person in representing himself/herself as Commission on Dietetic Registration credentialed when he/she is not.

17. The dietetics practitioner withdraws from professional practice under the following circumstances:

   a. The dietetics practitioner has engaged in any substance abuse that could affect his/her practice;

   b. The dietetics practitioner has been adjudged by a court to be mentally incompetent;

   c. The dietetics practitioner has an emotional or mental disability that affects his/her practice in a manner that could harm the client or others.

18. The dietetics practitioner complies with all applicable laws and regulations concerning the profession and is subject to disciplinary action under the following circumstances:

   a. The dietetics practitioner has been convicted of a crime under the laws of the United States which is a felony or a misdemeanor, an essential element of which is dishonesty, and which is related to the practice of the profession.

   b. The dietetics practitioner has been disciplined by a state, and at least one of the grounds for the discipline is the same or substantially equivalent to these principles.

   c. The dietetics practitioner has committed an act of misfeasance or malfeasance which is directly related to the practice of the profession as determined by a court of competent jurisdiction, a licensing board, or an agency of a governmental body.

19. The dietetics practitioner supports and promotes high standards of professional practice. The dietetics practitioner accepts the obligation to protect clients, the public, and the profession by upholding the Code of Ethics for the Profession of Dietetics and by reporting alleged violations of the Code through the defined review process of The American Dietetic Association and its credentialing agency, the Commission on Dietetic Registration.

Source: ADA. "Code of Ethics for the Profession of Dietetics." *J Am Diet Assoc* 99, no. 1(1999): 109–110.

Article II
of the Bylaws of the American
Dietetic Association

MEMBERS

Section 1. Classes of Members. The Association shall have the following five (5) classes of members:

Active   Retired   Student   Honorary   International

Section 2. Active Members. Qualifications.

2a. An individual holding a baccalaureate degree from a regionally accredited college or university, and meeting the academic requirements specified by Association; and one or more of the following criteria may apply for Active membership:
1. a Registered Dietitian ("RD") credentialed by the Commission on Dietetic Registration ("CDR");
2. has completed an academic and/or supervised practice program accredited by the Commission on Accreditation for Dietetics Education ("CADE");

2b. An individual holding a master's or a doctoral degree, and a degree (baccalaureate, master's, doctoral) in one of the following areas may apply for Active membership: dietetics, foods and nutrition, nutrition, community/public health nutrition, food science, or food service systems management. A regionally accredited college or university must have conferred each degree.

2c. An individual meeting one or more of the following criteria may apply for Active membership:

239

    1. a Dietetic Technician, Registered ("DTR") credentialed by the CDR or
       has established eligibility to take the examination for dietetic technicians;
    2. has completed a CADE approved associate degree program for dietetic
       technicians;
    3. holds a baccalaureate degree and meets the academic requirements spec-
       ified by CADE, and has completed a CADE accredited/approved dietetic
       technician program experience.

2d. An individual who previously paid the optional one-time dues in order to
obtain "life" membership in the Association, or has completed a term as
President of the Association.

Section 3. Retired Members. Qualifications. Any member of Association that
is no longer employed or actively engaged in dietetic practice or education and is
at least sixty-two (62) years of age, or is retired on total (permanent) disability
may apply for Retired membership.

Section 4. Student Members. Qualifications. Student classification can be held
for a maximum of six (6) years. An individual meeting one of the following criteria may apply for Student membership:

4a. A student enrolled in a CADE accredited/approved program;

4b. A student in a regionally accredited college or university who states his/her
intent to enter a CADE accredited/approved program;

4c. Active members returning to school on a full-time basis for a baccalaureate
or graduate degree in a dietetic related course of study may apply for Student membership status.

Section 5. Honorary Members. Qualifications. An individual who has made a
notable contribution to the field of nutrition and dietetics may be admitted to the
Association as an Honorary member upon invitation of the Board of Directors.

Section 6. International Members. Qualifications. An individual who has
completed formal training in food, nutrition or dietetics received outside the
United States and US Territories verified by the country's professional dietetics
association and/or country's regulatory body.

Section 7. Privileges of Membership.

Source: ADA. "Bylaws of American Association." www.eatright.org/Public/Other/index_
bylaws.cfw (accessed September 5, 2003): 1–4.

APPENDIX C

The American Dietetic Association Standards of Professional Practice for Dietetics Professionals

STANDARD 1: PROVISION OF SERVICES

Develops, implements, and promotes quality service based on client expectations and needs

Rationale

Dietetics professionals provide, facilitate, and promote quality services based on client needs and expectations, current knowledge, and professional experience.

Indicators

Each dietetics professional:

1.1 collaborates with client to assess needs, background, and resources and to establish mutual goals
1.2 collaborates with other professionals as appropriate
1.3 applies knowledge and skills to determine the most appropriate action plan
1.4 implements quality practice by following policies, procedures, legislation, licensure, practice guidelines, and the Standards of Professional Practice
1.5 fosters excellence and exhibits professionalism in practice
1.6 continuously evaluates processes and outcomes

1.7 advocates for the provision of food and nutrition services as part of public policy

Examples of Outcomes

- Clients actively participate in establishing goals and objectives
- Clients' needs are met
- Clients are satisfied with service and products provided
- Evaluation reflects expected outcomes
- Public has access to food and nutrition services

STANDARD 2: APPLICATION OF RESEARCH

Effectively applies, participates in, or generates research to enhance practice

Rationale

Effective application, support, and generation of dietetics research in practice encourages continuous quality improvement and provides documented support for the benefit of the client.

Indicators

Each dietetics professional:

2.1 locates and reviews research findings for their application to dietetics practice
2.2 bases practice on sound scientific principles, research, and theory
2.3 promotes research through alliances and collaboration with dietetics and other professionals and organizations
2.4 contributes to the development of new knowledge and research in dietetics
2.5 collects measurable data and documents outcomes within the practice setting
2.6 shares research data and activities through various media

Examples of Outcomes

- Client receives appropriate services based on the effective application of research
- A foundation for performance measurement and improvement is provided

- Outcomes data support reimbursement for the services of dietetics professionals
- Research findings are used for the development and revision of policies, procedures, practice guidelines, protocols, and clinical pathways
- Professionals use benchmarking and knowledge of "best practices" to improve performance

STANDARD 3: COMMUNICATION AND APPLICATION OF KNOWLEDGE

Successful dietetics professionals apply knowledge and communicate effectively with others

Rationale

Dietetics professionals work with and through others while using their unique knowledge of food, human nutrition, and management as well as skills in providing services.

Indicators

Each dietetics professional:

3.1 has knowledge related to a specific area(s) of professional service
3.2 communicates sound scientific principles, research, and theory
3.3 integrates knowledge of food and human nutrition with knowledge of health, social sciences, communication, and management theory
3.4 shares knowledge and information with clients
3.5 helps students and clients apply knowledge and skills
3.6 documents interpretation of relevant information and results of communication with professionals, personnel, students, or clients
3.7 contributes to the development of new knowledge
3.8 seeks out information to provide effective services

Examples of Outcomes

- Professional provides expertise in food, nutrition, and management information

- Client understands the information received
- Client receives current and appropriate information and knowledge
- Client knows how to obtain additional guidance

STANDARD 4: UTILIZATION AND MANAGEMENT OF RESOURCES

Uses resources effectively and efficiently in practice

Rationale

Appropriate use of time, money, facilities, and human resources facilitates delivery of quality services.

Indicators

Each dietetics professional:

4.1 uses a systematic approach to maintain and manage professional resources successfully

4.2 uses measurable resources such as personnel, monies, equipment, guidelines, protocols, reference materials, and time in the provision of dietetics services

4.3 analyzes safety, effectiveness, and cost in planning and delivering services and products

4.4 justifies use of resources by documenting consistency with plan, continuous quality improvement, and desired outcomes

4.5 educates and helps clients and others to identify and secure appropriate and available resources and services

Examples of Outcomes

- The dietetics professional documents use of resources according to plan and budget
- Resources and services are measured and data are used to promote and validate the effectiveness of services
- Desired outcomes are achieved and documented
- Resources are managed and used cost-effectively

STANDARD 5: QUALITY IN PRACTICE

Systematically evaluates the quality and effectiveness of practice and revises practice as needed to incorporate the results of evaluation

Rationale

Quality practice requires regular performance evaluation and continuous improvement of services.

Indicators

Each dietetics professional:

5.1 identifies performance improvement criteria to monitor effectiveness of services

5.2 identifies expected outcomes

5.3 documents outcomes of services provided

5.4 compares actual performance to expected outcomes

5.5 documents action taken when discrepancies exist between actual performance and expected outcomes

5.6 continuously evaluates and refines services based on measured outcomes

Examples of Outcomes

- Performance improvement criteria are measured
- Actual performance is evaluated
- Clients' outcomes meet established criteria (objectives/goals)
- Results of quality improvement activities direct refinement of practice

STANDARD 6: CONTINUED COMPETENCE AND PROFESSIONAL ACCOUNTABILITY

Engages in lifelong self-development to improve knowledge and skills that promote continued competence

Rationale

Professional practice requires continuous acquisition of knowledge and skill development to maintain accountability to the public.

Indicators

Each dietetics professional:

6.1 conducts self-assessment at regular intervals to identify professional strengths and weaknesses

6.2 identifies needs for professional development and mentors others

6.3 develops and implements a plan for professional growth

6.4 documents professional development activities

6.5 adheres to the Code of Ethics for the profession of dietetics and is accountable and responsible for actions and behavior

6.6 supports the application of research findings to professional practice

6.7 takes active leadership roles

Examples of Outcomes

- Dietetics professional uses self-reflection and feedback from a variety of sources to evaluate and implement professional change
- Dietetics professional development needs are identified and directed learning takes place
- Dietetics professional accepts accountability to the public
- Dietetics professional obtains appropriate certifications
- Dietetics professional supports legislation which promotes positive food and nutrition outcomes
- Dietetics professional uses "best practices" to demonstrate competency
- Dietetics professional meets Commission on Dietetic Registration recertification requirements

Source: ADA. "The American Dietetic Association Standards of Professional Practice for Dietetics Professionals." *J Am Diet Assoc* 98, no. 1 (1998): 84–85.

APPENDIX D

Position Paper Update for 2004

FOOD CHOICES

- Total diet approach to communicate food and nutrition information. *J Am Diet Assoc.* 2002;102:100. (Expires 2006)
- Vegetarian diets. *J Am Diet Assoc.* 2002;103:749. (Expires 2007) ADA and Dietitians of Canada Joint Position. Also see: A new food guide for North American vegetarians. *J Am Diet Assoc.* 2003;103:771.
- Health implications of dietary fiber. *J Am Diet Assoc.* 2002;102:993. (Expires 2007)
- Functional foods. *J Am Diet Assoc.* 1999;99:1278. (Reaffirmed—an update will be published in 2004.)
- Food fortification and dietary supplements. *J Am Diet Assoc.* 2001;101: 115. (Expires December 31, 2004)
- Position paper on trans-fatty acids. (American Society of Clinical Nutrition/American Institute of Nutrition). *J Am Diet Assoc.* 1996. (Not reprinted in *J Am Diet Assoc.* Originally published in the *Am J Clin Nutr.* 1996;63: 663.) This will be replaced after the approval and publication of a new position "Dietary fatty acids" in 2004.

FOOD SUPPLY

Safety

- Food and water safety. *J Am Diet Assoc.* 2003;103:1203. (Expires 2007)

Supplementation/Fortification

- The impact of fluoride on health. Complete version, *J Am Diet Assoc.* 2000; 100:1208. (Reaffirmed; an update will be published in 2005) [Reprinted with missing figures in January 2001, *J Am Diet Assoc.* 2001;101:126.]

Substitutes

- Fat replacers. *J Am Diet Assoc.* 1998; 98:463. (Reaffirmed—an update position will be published in 2005)
- Use of nutritive and nonnutritive sweeteners. *J Am Diet Assoc.* 1998; 98:580. (Reaffirmed—an update will be published in 2004)

Food Security/Environment

- Biotechnology and the future of food. *J Am Diet Assoc.* 1995;95:1429. (Reaffirmed—an update position will be published in 2004.)
- Domestic food and nutrition security. *J Am Diet Assoc.* 2002;102:1840. (Expires 2005)
- Dietetics professionals can implement practices to conserve natural resources and protect the environment. *J Am Diet Assoc.* 2001;101:1221. (Expires 2006)
- Addressing world hunger, malnutrition, and food insecurity. *J Am Diet Assoc.* 2003;103:1046. (Expires 2008)

LIFE SPAN

Pregnancy/Breastfeeding

- Breaking the barriers to breastfeeding. *J Am Diet Assoc.* 2001;101:1213. (Reaffirmed—an update will be published in 2005)
- Nutrition and lifestyle for a healthy pregnancy outcome. *J Am Diet Assoc.* 2002;102:1479. (Expires 2007)
- ADA supports National Association of WIC Directors position on breastfeeding promotion in the WIC program. (Revised 1994) *J Am Diet Assoc.* 1990;90:8. (Not reprinted in *J Am Diet Assoc.*)

Infancy/Childhood

- Child and adolescent food and nutrition programs. *J Am Diet Assoc.* 2003;103:887. (Expires 2006)
- Dietary guidance for healthy children ages 2–11 years. *J Am Diet Assoc.* 1999;98:93 (Reaffirmed—an update will be published in 2004)
- Local support for nutrition integrity in schools. *J Am Diet Assoc.* 2000;100:108. (Expires 2005)
- Nutrition standards for child care programs. *J Am Diet Assoc.* 1999;99: 981. (Reaffirmed—an update will be published in 2005)
- Nutrition services: an essential component of comprehensive school health programs. *J Am Diet Assoc.* 2003;102:505. (Expires 2008) ADA, American School Food Service Association and Society for Nutrition Education Joint Position.

Adults

- Nutrition and athletic performance for adults. *J Am Diet Assoc.* 2000; 100:1543. (Expires 2005) ADA, Dietitians of Canada and American College of Sports Medicine Joint Position.
- Women's health and nutrition. *J Am Diet Assoc.* 1999;99:738. (Reaffirmed—an update will be published in 2004) ADA Dietitians of Canada Joint Position.

Elderly

- Liberalized diets for older adults in long term care. *J Am Diet Assoc.* 2002;102:1316. (Expires 2005)
- Nutrition, aging and the continuum of care. *J Am Diet Assoc.* 2000;100:580 (Reaffirmed—an update will be published in 2004)

NUTRITION MANAGEMENT

Disease/Special Conditions

- Nutrition intervention in the treatment of anorexia nervosa, bulimia nervosa, and eating disorders not otherwise specified (EDNOS). *J Am Diet Assoc.* 2001;101:810. (Expires 2006)

- Nutrition intervention in the care of persons with human immunodeficiency virus infection. *J Am Diet Assoc.* 2000;100:708. (Reaffirmed—an update will be published in 2004) ADA and Dietitians of Canada Joint Position.
- Providing nutrition services for infants, children, and adults with development disabilities and special health care needs. *J Am Diet Assoc.* 2004;104: 97–107.
- Ethical and legal issues in nutrition, hydration, and feeding. *J Am Diet Assoc.* 2002;102:716. (Expires 2007)

MNT/Health Care

- Integration of Medical Nutrition Therapy and Pharmacotherapy. *J Am Diet Assoc.* 2003;103:1363. (Expires 2007)
- Cost-effectiveness of Medical Nutrition Therapy. *J Am Diet Assoc.* 1995;95:88. (Reaffirmed—an update will be published in 2004)
- Nutrition services in managed care. *J Am Diet Assoc.* 2002;102:1471. (Expires 2005)

Weight Management

- Weight management. *J Am Diet Assoc.* 2002;102:1145. (Expires 2006)

PUBLIC HEALTH

- Oral health and nutrition. *J Am Diet Assoc.* 2003;103:615. (Expires 2006)
- Role of the dietetics professionals in health promotion and disease prevention programs. *J Am Diet Assoc.* 2002;102:1680. (Expires 2005)
- Food and nutrition misinformation. *J Am Diet Assoc.* 2002;102:260. (Expires 2005)

Accessing ADA Positions

Positions are available for viewing or downloading from the ADA Web site at *http://www.eatright.org/Public/index_7705.cfm.* Single copies of positions can be mailed or faxed upon request. Contact ADA Headquarters (800/877-1600, ext. 4892 or e-mail *ppapers@eatright.org*). The complete collection of positions is available for purchase through the ADA member service center (312/899-0040, ext. 5000) or may be ordered from the ADA Catalog of Products and Services (catalog number 0671).

Contact Cathy Devlin, RD, at ADA Headquarters (800/877-1600, ext. 4835 or e-mail, *cdevlin@eatright.org*) for answers to your questions on ADA positions.

FANSA STATEMENTS

The Food and Nutrition Science Alliance (FANSA) is a partnership of four professional scientific societies (ADA, the American Society for Clinical Nutrition, the American Society for Nutritional Sciences, and the Institute of Food Technologists) whose members have joined forces to speak with one voice on food and nutrition science issues.

FANSA'a combined membership includes more than 100,000 food, nutrition, and medical practitioners and scientists. Copies of FANSA statements may be viewed and downloaded at http://www.eatright.org/Public/index_7705.cfm. Single copies are available by contacting ADA headquarters (ppapers@eatright.org or 800/877-1600, ext 4892).

Current FANSA statements are:

- Folic Acid: A reminder for women before and during pregnancy. (Released October 1995)
- What does the public need to know about dietary supplements? (Released June 1997; published in *J Am Diet Assoc*. 1997; 97:728)
- Making sense of scientific research about diet and health. (Released August 1997)
- Making sense of risks associated with diets. (Released September 1997)
- Diet and cancer prevention in the United States. (Released December 1999)
- What consumers need to know about vitamin E. (Released August 2000)

Source: ADA. "Position Paper Update for 2004." *J Am Diet Assoc* 104, no. 2(2004): 276–278.

Accreditation Standards for Entry-Level Education Programs

CADE accredits programs by evaluating their compliance with the accreditation standards for entry-level dietetics education programs. Each of the three standards consists of a principle, statements describing CADE expectations, and examples of evidence that can be used to document how well the program meets the standard.

Principles are comprehensive statements of ideals that are held true and serve as the foundation and rationale for standards. The standards statements are requirements and serve as the basis for both internal and external program evaluations. Examples of evidence illustrate the type of documentation that may be appropriate for the self-study report, for distance education programs, for new programs, and for programs preparing for a site visit. Examples of evidence are intended as guidelines only and are not all-inclusive.

STANDARD ONE: PROGRAM PLANNING AND OUTCOMES ASSESSMENT

Principle

Philosophical premises underlie the establishment and nature of any planned program. This philosophical basis is formalized in the program mission and determines the goals to which a program is directed. Identification, articulation, and on-going examination of the mission and goals of an educational program enable the program to develop and progress in an efficient, planned manner. Systematic and continuous internal and external evaluation of relevant outcomes provides necessary feedback to ensure that program goals continue to be appropriate and that goals are attained.

Standard One

The dietetics education program has clearly defined a mission, goals, program outcomes, and assessment measures and implements a systematic, continuous process to assess outcomes, evaluate goal achievement, and improve program effectiveness.

- The program has established a mission and demonstrates that the mission is compatible with the mission statement or philosophy of the sponsoring organization and the preparation of entry-level dietetics practitioners.
- The program has established goals and demonstrates how these goals reflect the program's mission statement and the environment in which the program exists.
- The program has established outcomes and appropriate measures to assess achievement of goals and program effectiveness, including at least program completion rates, postgraduate performance, such as supervised practice program placement, job placement, or graduate school acceptance rates, and the pass rate of first-time test takers on the registration examination. If the pass rate is less than 80 percent for first-time test takers, the program implements and monitors a plan of action to improve graduate performance.
- The program demonstrates that administrators, faculty/preceptors, students, graduates, individuals outside the program, and other appropriate constituencies participate in a systematic process of planning, implementation, and evaluation, on a regular and continuing basis, of all components of the program and its effectiveness.
- The program demonstrates that its planning and evaluation process includes evidence that data are collected and analyzed to identify the extent that goals for the program are being achieved and feedback is incorporated to improve the program.
- Through the evaluation process, the program has identified strengths and limitations and has delineated short- and long-term plans for management of the program to assist in achieving program goals.

STANDARD TWO: CURRICULUM AND STUDENT LEARNING OUTCOMES

Principle

An entry-level dietetics education program is based on knowledge, skills, and competencies necessary to provide dietetics services. The curriculum sequentially builds knowledge, skills, and competencies for each student. Graduates must demonstrate the ability to communicate, collaborate, work in teams to solve problems, and apply critical thinking skills. The curriculum will vary with the program environment, the type of program, mission, goals, measurable outcomes for the program, and student needs.

Standard Two

The dietetics education program has a planned curriculum that provides for achievement of student learning outcomes and expected competence of the graduate.

- The program demonstrates that the curriculum is based on the foundation knowledge and skills and/or competencies defined for an entry-level dietetic technician or dietitian according to the type of program (see Sections III and IV, pages 29–35 and 37–41).
  - The CP curriculum is based on the Foundation Knowledge and Skills and Competency Statements for dietitians
  - The DPD curriculum is based on the Foundation Knowledge and Skills Statements for dietitians
  - The DI curriculum is based on the Competency Statements for dietitians
  - The DT curriculum is based on the Foundation Knowledge and Skills and Competency Statements for dietetic technicians
- The program demonstrates how the curriculum is consistent with the mission, goals, and measurable outcomes for the program.
- The program demonstrates that the curriculum includes both didactic and practice-related learning experiences according to the type of program.
- The CP and DI programs demonstrate that the curriculum includes a minimum of one emphasis area in addition to the core competencies. To accomplish the foregoing, the program chooses from the following options and is able to justify its choice(s) on the basis of mission, goals, and resources:
  - Uses one or more of the four defined emphasis areas;
  - Develops a general emphasis area by selecting a minimum of seven competency statements, with at least one from each of the four defined emphasis areas;

- Creates a unique emphasis area, with a minimum of seven competency statements, based on local resources and identified needs.
- The program demonstrates that the curriculum logically progresses from introductory learning experiences to the expected learning outcomes upon completion of the program (novice to beginner to competent).
- The program demonstrates use of a variety of educational approaches (e.g., field trips, role-playing, simulations, problem-based learning, distance education, classroom instruction, and laboratory experiences) to facilitate student learning outcomes.
- The program implements an assessment process to demonstrate that learning experiences develop communication, collaboration, teamwork, problem solving, and critical thinking skills.
- The program implements an assessment process to demonstrate that learning opportunities develop personal and professional attitudes and values, ethical practice, and leadership and decision-making skills.
- The program demonstrates that the curriculum includes experiences with other disciplines and exposure to a variety of dietetics practice settings, individuals, and groups.
- The program demonstrates that curriculum length is based on the program mission and goals, conforms to commonly accepted practice in higher education, and is consistent with student learning outcomes.
- The CP, DI, and DT programs demonstrate that the supervised practice experiences are directly related to the planned curriculum.
- The program implements a process to assess student progress toward achievement of student learning outcomes, using a variety of methods during and at the conclusion of the program.
- The program demonstrates periodic evaluation of the curriculum objectives, content, length, and educational methods, to improve educational quality. Periodic evaluation includes assessment of new knowledge and technology impacting dietetics practice.
- The program demonstrates use of a process to monitor the comparability of educational experiences and of evaluation strategies used to assess student progress, and it ensures consistency of learning outcomes when students are assigned to different sites for the same type of experiences.

STANDARD THREE: PROGRAM MANAGEMENT

Principle

An education program requires sound management of all components, including the resources necessary for effective education to occur. Resources include competent and sufficient program administrators, faculty and/or preceptors, support personnel, and adequate services to provide for the planned education of students. Fair, equitable, and considerate treatment of both prospective students and those enrolled in the educational program is incorporated into all aspects of the program.

Standard Three

Management of the dietetics education program and availability of program resources are evident in defined processes and procedures and demonstrate accountability to students and the public.

- The program demonstrates that the program director has the authority, responsibility, and sufficient time to manage the program, including assessment, planning, implementation, and evaluation critical for program effectiveness. Program director responsibilities include at least
  - policy development;
  - student recruitment, advisement, evaluation, and counseling;
  - program record maintenance, including student complaints and resolutions;
  - curriculum development;
  - program communication and coordination;
  - continuous internal and external program evaluation.
- The program demonstrates that it has the administrative and financial support, learning resources, physical facilities, and support services needed to accomplish its goals. The annual budget for the program or other financial information, such as percentage of department budget allocated to support the program, is sufficient to produce the desired outcomes.
- The program demonstrates that it has a sufficient number of faculty and/or preceptors to provide learning experiences and exposure to the diversity of practice. Faculty and/or preceptors can show evidence of continued competency appropriate to teaching responsibilities, through professional work experience, graduate education, continuing education, research, or other activities leading to professional growth and the advancement of their profession. In addition,
  - Faculty in regionally accredited colleges and universities meet the institution's criteria for appointment.
  - Preceptors in supervised practice programs are credentialed or licensed as appropriate for the area in which they are supervising students or demonstrate equivalent education and experience.
- The CP, DI, and DT programs demonstrate that a process is used to select and periodically evaluate adequacy and appropriateness of facilities, to pro-

vide supervised practice learning experiences compatible with the competencies students are expected to achieve.

- The CP, DI, and DT programs demonstrate that a process is used to maintain written agreements, signed by administrators with appropriate authority and delineating the responsibility between the sponsoring organization and affiliating institutions, organizations, and/or agencies providing supervised practice experiences.
- The program provides clear, consistent, and truthful information to prospective students, enrolled students, and the public at large. Program information is accessible in a catalog, program bulletin, brochure, or other printed and/or electronic materials. Program information includes at least the following:
  - Type and description of the program, including mission, goals, and measurable outcomes
  - Description of how the program fits into the credentialing process for dietetics practitioners
  - Cost to student, such as estimated expenses for travel, housing, books, liability insurance, medical exams, and uniforms, in addition to application fees and tuition, if applicable
  - Accreditation status, including the full name, address, and phone number of CADE
  - Admission requirements
  - Academic/program calendar or schedule
  - Graduation and/or program completion requirements
  - Computer matching information (for DI programs, if applicable)
- The program protects student civil rights and complies with institutional equal opportunity programs.
- The program makes students aware of and implements written policies and procedures that protect the rights of students and are consistent with current institutional practice. Policies and procedures include at least the following:
  - Withdrawal and refund of tuition and fees
  - Scheduling and program calendar, including vacation and holidays
  - Protection of privacy of information
  - Access to personal files
  - Access to student support services, including health services, counseling and testing, and financial aid resources
  - Insurance requirements, including those for professional liability
  - Liability for safety in travel to or from assigned areas
  - Injury or illness while in a facility for supervised practice
  - Grievance procedures
  - Assessment of prior learning and credit toward program requirements (coursework and/or experiential)

- Formal assessment of student learning and regular reports of performance and progress at specified intervals throughout the program, such as within and at the conclusion of any given course, unit, segment, or rotation of a planned learning experience
- Disciplinary/termination procedures
- Graduation and/or program completion requirements, including guidelines ensuring that all students completing requirements as established by the program receive verification statements

Source: ADA. Accreditation Handbook, 2002. Commission on Accreditation for Dietetics Education.

Standards of Professional Practices for Dietetics Professionals in Management and Foodservice Settings

BRIDGET GRIFFIN, MPH, RD; JANE M. DUNN, MS, RD; JILL IRVIN, MA, RD; INEZ F. SPERANZA, RD

STANDARD 1: PROVISION OF SERVICES

Provides quality service based on expectations and needs of clients/customers

Rationale

Management professionals provide, facilitate, and promote quality service based on client/customer needs and expectations, current knowledge of food service practices, and professional experience.

Indicators

Each management professional:

1.1 collaborates with client/customer to assess needs, backgrounds, and resources and to establish mutual goals, which are consistent with the mission and vision of the organization;

1.2 collaborates with others;

1.3 applies knowledge and skills to determine the most appropriate plan;

1.4 identifies advantages of client's/customer's expertise;

1.5 implements quality practice by following policies, procedures, legislation and regulation, licensure, practice guidelines, accreditation standards, and the Standards of Professional Practice;

1.6 determines quality improvement initiatives, evaluates data and findings, and assures that performance improvement is implemented;

1.7 participates in achieving the goals of the facility/client.

Examples of Outcomes

- Client/customer needs are used as the basis for establishing goals and objectives.
- Clients/customers indicate/express satisfaction with service and products provided.
- Service and program evaluations indicate overall achievement of client/customer expectations.
- Opportunities to improve services and programs to meet/ exceed client/customer expectations are addressed.
- Public accesses food and nutrition services.

STANDARD 2: APPLICATION OF RESEARCH

Effectively applies, participates in, or generates research to enhance practice

Rationale

Effective application, support, and generation of dietetics research in practice encourage continuous quality improvement and provide documented support for the benefit of the client/customer.

Indicators

Each management professional:

2.1 bases practice on sound scientific principles, research, and theory;

2.2 promotes research through alliances and collaboration with management and other professionals and organizations;

2.3 collaborates with other research sources to identify research objectives;

2.4 contributes to the development of new knowledge and research in management;

2.5 collects measurable data and documents outcomes within the business setting;

2.6 shares research data and activities through various media;

2.7 locates, reviews, and supports the application of research findings to management practice.

Examples of Outcomes

- Management professional effectively applies research in providing services to the client/customer.
- Management professional establishes a foundation for performance measurement, and improvement is documented.
- Management professional provides outcomes data, which demonstrate the cost-effectiveness of services provided.
- Management professional uses research findings for the development, evaluation, and revision of services and products.
- Management professional uses benchmarking and knowledge of "best practices" to improve performance.

STANDARD 3: COMMUNICATION AND APPLICATION OF KNOWLEDGE

Effectively applies knowledge and communicates with others

Rationale

Management professionals work with and through others using their unique knowledge of food, human nutrition, and management, as well as skills in providing services.

Indicators

Each management professional:

3.1 communicates current sound principles, research, and theory;

3.2 integrates and communicates management theory with knowledge of food and human nutrition as well as health and social sciences;

3.3 guides clients/customers in applying knowledge and skills;

3.4 documents interpretation of relevant information and results of communication with clients/customers;

3.5 manages information services to support effective and efficient provision of products and services.

Examples of Outcomes

- Management professional demonstrates expertise in the management of food and nutrition systems.
- Management professional aggregates and/or presents data or concepts to individuals or boards responsible for making policy.
- Client/customer receives current and appropriate information.
- Client/customer communicates understanding of and demonstrates the application of information received.
- Client/customer acknowledges management professional as source of accurate and reliable information.

STANDARD 4: UTILIZATION AND MANAGEMENT OF RESOURCES

Uses resources effectively and efficiently in practice

Rationale

Appropriate use of time, money, facilities, and human resources facilitates delivery of quality services.

Indicators

Each management professional:

4.1 uses a systematic approach to obtain, maintain, and manage resources successfully;

4.2 uses measurable resources such as personnel, money, equipment, materials, and time effectively in the provision of services;

4.3 analyzes market conditions, effectiveness, quality, safety, and cost in planning and delivering of services and products

4.4 informs and advises others to identify and secure appropriate and available resources and services.

Examples of Outcomes

- Management professional measures resources and services and uses data to promote and validate the effectiveness of services.
- Management professional achieves business plans and documents success.
- Management professional utilizes resources in a cost-effective manner.
- Management professional identifies and employs best practices in culinary techniques.
- Management professional implements and maintains a superior food safety program.
- Management professional educates and trains personnel to do their job to the best of their abilities.
- Management professional creates partnerships with suppliers, which are ethical and mutually beneficial.
- Management professional identifies costs and benefits of importing expertise.
- Management professional develops and supports effective teams in a culturally diverse work force.

STANDARD 5: QUALITY IN PRACTICE

Systematically evaluates the quality and effectiveness of practice and revises practice as needed to incorporate the results of evaluation

Rationale

Quality practice requires regular performance evaluation and continuous improvement of services.

Indicators

Each management professional:

5.1 identifies expected outcomes;
5.2 documents outcomes of services provided;

5.3 compares actual performance to expected outcomes;

5.4 documents action taken when discrepancies exist between actual performance and expected outcomes;

5.5 continuously evaluates and improves services based on measured outcomes;

5.6 maintains knowledge of and compliance with standards as mandated by regulatory agencies.

Examples of Outcomes

- Management professional establishes performance improvement processes and criteria.
- Management professional evaluates actual performance of services and programs, using established criteria.
- Outcomes meet established criteria (objectives/goals/ business plans).
- Management professional uses results of quality improvement activities to direct refinement of services and programs.
- Financial reports, such as profit and loss and percent participation, document efficiency and cost-effectiveness.
- Management professional ensures the safety of all food and nutrition products served to clients/customers.

STANDARD 6: CONTINUED COMPETENCE AND PROFESSIONAL ACCOUNTABILITY

Engages in lifelong self-development to improve knowledge and enhance professional competence

Rationale

Professional practice requires continuous acquisition of knowledge and skill development to maintain accountability to the public.

Indicators

Each management professional:

6.1 conducts self-assessment at regular intervals to identify professional strengths and weaknesses;

6.2 identifies needs for professional development and mentors others;

6.3 develops and implements a plan for professional growth;

6.4 documents professional development activities;

6.5 adheres to the Code of Ethics for the profession of dietetics and is accountable and responsible for actions and behavior;

6.6 takes active leadership roles;

6.7 advocates for the provision of food and nutrition services;

6.8 embraces opportunities to remain on the cutting edge of management practice.

Examples of Outcomes

- Management professional uses self-reflection and feedback from a variety of sources to evaluate and implement professional change.
- Management professional identifies, seeks, and completes learning based on a plan for professional growth.
- Management professional accepts accountability to the public.
- Management professional obtains appropriate certifications.
- Management professional supports legislation which promotes positive food and nutrition outcomes.
- Management professional uses "best practices" to demonstrate competency.
- Management professional meets Commission on Dietetic Registration recertification requirements.
- Management professional mentors students and colleagues.
- Management professional nurtures networks with other directors and management professionals.

Approved by the ADA Quality Management Committee in October 2000. Approved by the Executive Committee of the Management in Food and Nutrition Systems dietetic practice group in March 2001.

Source: Griffin, Bridget, Jane M. Dunn, Jill Irvin, and Inez F. Speranza. "Standards of Professional Practices for Dietetics Professionals in Management and Foodservice Settings." *J Am Diet Assoc* 101, no. 8(2001): 944–946.

Standards of Professional Practice: Measuring the Beliefs and Realities of Consultant Dietitians in Health Care Facilities

JODY LYNN VOGELZANG, MS, RD, FADA;
LORI LYNN ROTH-YOUSEY, MPH, RD

STANDARD 1: PROVISION OF SERVICES

Provides quality service based on clients' expectations and needs.

Rationale

Dietetics professionals provide, facilitate, and promote quality services based on client needs and expectations, organizational structure of work environment, current knowledge, and professional experience.

Indicators

Each dietetics professional:

1.1 collaborates and establishes mutual goals with clients by assessing needs, background, and resources
1.2 collaborates with other professionals, as appropriate

1.3 applies knowledge and skills to determine the most appropriate action plan

1.4 implements quality practice by following policies, procedures, Federal/State legislation, licensure, practice guidelines, medical nutrition therapy protocols (MNT) and the Standards of Professional Practice

1.5 fosters excellence and exhibits professionalism in practice

1.6 continuously evaluates processes and outcomes

1.7 advocates for the provision of food and nutrition services as part of public policy

Examples of Outcomes

- Dietetics professional meets client needs and is aware of communication effectiveness.
- Clients are satisfied with provided services and products.
- Client-centered goals are individualized and protect confidentiality rights.
- Dietetics professional initiates or participates in advocacy by: identifying a problem needing public attention, speaking or writing about a problem to bring attention toward a potential policy, or helping to draft information to be used in public policy formation. Examples of policy elements related to CD-HCF are providing adequate food for populations at a reasonable cost, ensuring food access and availability, integrating nutrition into the health care system, and population-specific medical nutrition therapy.

STANDARD 2: APPLICATION OF RESEARCH

Effectively applies, supports, and participates in dietetics research to enhance practice

Rationale

Effective application of, support for and participation in dietetics research encourages continuous quality improvement and documents benefits for clients.

Indicators

Each dietetics professional:

2.1 reviews research findings for their application

2.2 bases practice on sound, scientific principles, research and theory

2.3 promotes research through combined collaborations with dietetics professionals, other business and health care professionals and non-profit and for-profit organizations

2.4.0 advances the development of new knowledge and dietetics research using training, experience, and work environment opportunities by:

2.4.1 collecting measurable data

2.4.2 documenting outcomes within the practice setting

2.4.3 evaluating outcomes resulting from client services

2.4.4 sharing research results (as appropriate) with clients using written reports, verbal communication and other media

Examples of Outcomes

- Clients receive appropriate services based on the effective application of research.
- Objective performance measures are monitored to identify service areas needing improvement.
- Dietetics professional uses benchmarking and knowledge of "best practices" to improve performance.
- Outcomes results benefit clients and support reimbursement for services provided by dietetics professional.
- Research contributions are used for the development and revision of policies, procedures, practice guidelines, protocols, and clinical pathways.
- Outcomes results are shared with clients using appropriate reports, presentations, mentoring, and various interactive teaching modalities (i.e., technology).
- Research findings are used to develop or revise public policy.

STANDARD 3: COMMUNICATION AND APPLICATION OF KNOWLEDGE

Applies food, human nutrition, and management knowledge and communicates with others

Rationale

Dietetics professionals work with and through others while using their unique knowledge and communication skills in providing services.

Indicators

Each dietetics professional:

3.1 has knowledge related to a specific area(s) of professional service (i.e., geriatric nutrition)

3.2 communicates sound, scientific principles, research, and theory

3.3 integrates knowledge of food and human nutrition with knowledge of health, social sciences, communication, and management theory

3.4 shares knowledge and information with clients

3.5 helps clients apply knowledge and skills

3.6 documents interpretation of relevant information and results of communication with professionals, personnel, students, or clients

3.7 mentors and/or collaborates with entry-level dietitians, other dietetic professionals, dietary managers, and dietetics students

3.8 mentors other entry-level management trainees, health care and business/management students, and other health care team members

3.9 provides effective services using up-to-date and appropriate information

Examples of Outcomes

- Dietetics professional provides expertise in food preparation, MNT, and practice management.
- Clients apply and/or demonstrate understanding of information received.
- Dietetics professional measures communication effectiveness by assessing clients' behaviors and organizational performance.
- Clients receive current and appropriate information and knowledge through effective communication.
- Students, trainees, or other multi-professional, multi-care team members within a facility or in the community develop knowledge and skills as a result of dietetics professional applying and sharing knowledge, expertise and time.

STANDARD 4: UTILIZATION AND MANAGEMENT OF RESOURCES

Uses resources effectively and efficiently in practice

Rationale

Appropriate use of measurable resources (i.e., time, money, business plan, facilities, food purchases, foodservice equipment, computer programs and equipment, medical nutrition therapy protocols, standards of care, human resources and ongoing nutrition personnel training) facilitates delivery of quality services.

Indicators

Each dietetics professional:

4.1 uses a systematic approach to successfully manage measurable resources
4.2 uses measurable resources in the provision of dietetics services
4.3 analyzes safety, effectiveness and cost in planning and delivering services and products
4.4 justifies use of resources by documenting consistency with plan, continuous quality improvement, and desired outcomes
4.5 educates clients to identify and secure appropriate and available resources

Examples of Outcomes

- Dietetics professional documents time worked in a facility (or facilities) or individual practice according to a plan and budget.
- Dietetics professional negotiates adequate time to promote and validate the effectiveness of services.
- Desired outcomes of clients are achieved and documented.
- Measured resources are cost-effectively applied while maintaining quality (i.e., food quality, service quality, ongoing education/training quality).

STANDARD 5: QUALITY IN PRACTICE

Systematically evaluates the quality and effectiveness of practice and revises practice as needed to incorporate the results of evaluation

Rationale

Quality practice requires regular performance evaluation and continuous improvement of services.

Indicators

Each dietetics professional:

5.1 identifies professional standards that constitute quality and objectively measures his/her own performance in relation to attaining the quality

5.2   identifies expected outcomes related to his/her professional consulting activities

5.3   documents outcomes of services provided

5.4   compares actual performance to expected outcomes

5.5   documents action taken when discrepancies exist between actual performance and expected outcomes

5.6   continuously evaluates and refines services based on measured processes and outcomes

Examples of Outcomes

- Dietetics professional identifies and develops nutrition-related goals and objectives that constitute quality for facilities he/she consults.
- Actual performance is documented and evaluated.
- Clients' outcomes and dietetics professional performance meet established criteria (goals/objectives).
- Results of quality improvement activities direct refinement of practice.

STANDARD 6: CONTINUED COMPETENCE AND PROFESSIONAL ACCOUNTABILITY

Engages in lifelong, self-development to improve knowledge and enhance professional competence

Rationale

Professional practice requires continuous acquisition of knowledge and skill development to maintain accountability to the public.

Indicators

Each dietetics professional:

6.1   conducts self-assessment at regular intervals to identify professional strengths and weaknesses

6.2   identifies needs for professional development

6.3   develops and implements a plan of professional growth

6.4   documents professional development activities

6.5 adheres to the Code of Ethics for the profession of dietetics and is accountable and responsible for actions and behavior

6.6 supports the application of research findings to professional practice

6.7 takes active leadership roles and mentors others

Examples of Outcomes

- Dietetics professional uses self-reflection and feedback from a variety of sources to evaluate and implement professional change.
- Dietetics professional identifies development needs and self-directs learning.
- Dietetics professional is accountable to clients.
- Dietetics professional obtains appropriate certifications.
- Dietetics professional provides legislative lobbying efforts promoting positive food and nutrition outcomes and level of support is dependent on training, availability, and time. Dietetics professional uses "best practices" to demonstrate competency.
- Dietetics professional meets Commission on Dietetic Registration credentialing requirements.
- Dietetics professional upholds accountability to clients or peer complaints.

Source: Vogelzang, Jody Lynn, and Lori Lynn Roth-Yousey. "Standards of Professional Practice: Measuring the Beliefs and Realities of Consultant Dietitians in Health Care Facilities," *J Am Diet Assoc* 101, no. 4 (2001): 473–480.

Index

informational roles of managers, 167
instruction design, 176–183
instructional materials, 181–183
instructional strategies, 179–181
instructors. *See* educators, dietitians as
insurance. *See* health insurance
International Congress of Dietetics, 13
international membership, ADA, 21
interpersonal skills, 160–162, 167, 175,
226
intervention, nutrition, 84
interviewing, 185, 188–190
intrapreneur, defined, 130

J
*JADA (Journal of the American Dietetic
Association)*, 7
jails. *See* long-term care, food services in
JCAHO (Joint Commission on
Accreditation of Health
Organizations), 73, 130
job instruction training, 179–181. *See also*
education in dietetics
job possibilities. *See* career possibilities
job settings. *See* employment settings
*Journal of the American Dietetic
Association*, 7

K
knowledge economy, 220

L
laboratory experiments, as teaching
method, 180
law, issues of. *See* legislative issues
LDs (licensed dietitians), 15. *See also*
licensure
leadership roles, 102–103, 155–168. *See
also* management in dietetics
attaining skills for, 157–159
competencies, 226
conceptual skills, 165–167
human relations, 160–162
technical skills, 162–164
learning. *See* education in dietetics
lecturing, as teaching method, 180
legislative issues, 10, 71–74

contracts, 72, 121
dietetic consultants, 122, 129
government research, 208
politics, 65–67
licensure, 9, 61. *See also* LDs
state laws, 72
lifelong professional development, 67–71,
137. *See also* education in
dietetics
listening skills, 160
long-range planning. *See* future of
dietetics
long-term care
consultancy in, 121–124
defined, 92, 130
food services in, 97–98
regulations affecting, 73

M
managed health care, 82, 92, 130
management in dietetics, 92, 155–168
AMFO (Association for Managers of
Food Operations), 10
clinical dietetics, 167
competencies, 160–167
dietary managers, 10
clinical nutrition managers, 88
education background, 47–49
food and nutrition systems, 95–105
areas of employment, 96–100, 104
functions of, 159, 167
leadership qualities, 102–103
roles and responsibilities, 100–102
marketing dietitian services, 126
networking, 135–136, 148, 162
Web site, establishing, 137
master of science (MS) degree, 50
Maternal and Child Health Bill, 10
maternal health specialists, 112
media specialists in public health, 112
medical education, dietetics as part of,
145. *See also* educators,
dietitians as
medical insurance. *See* health insurance
medical nutrition therapy, 84–86
Medicare, 122, 130
membership in ADA, 9, 21–23